WP LIFE SERIES 4

lower blood pressure
LOWER
CHOLESTEROL

Catherine Butterfield

About the author

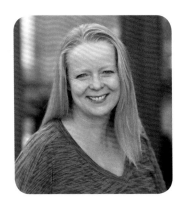

Catherine Butterfield was an award-winning print journalist before taking a career detour into health public relations. Working at some of Australia's largest hospitals alongside world-leading medical specialists, Catherine developed a keen interest in all things health-related. When she left the hospital setting to start a family, Catherine resumed writing and established a successful freelance writing business, Write Away Media. She has regularly contributed to Australian daily newspapers' custom publications, including *The Age* and *The Sydney Morning Herald*, magazines including the Royal Botanic Gardens publication and has a number of commercial publications to her name. *Lower Blood Pressure Lower Cholesterol* is Catherine's first book with Wilkinson Publishing.

Published by
Wilkinson Publishing Pty Ltd
ACN 006 042 173
Level 4, 2 Collins Street, Melbourne, Vic 3000
Tel: 03 9654 5446 www.wilkinsonpublishing.com.au

National Library of Australia Cataloguing-in-Publication entry:

Author:	Butterfield, Catherine, author.
Title:	Lower blood pressure lower cholesterol / Catherine Butterfield.
ISBN:	9781922178367 (paperback)
Subjects:	Cardiovascular system--Diseases--Risk factors.
	Cardiovascular system--Diseases--Prevention.
	Cardiovascular system--Diseases--Treatment.
	Heart--Diseases--Risk factors.
	Heart--Diseases--Prevention.
	Heart--Diseases--Treatment.
	Hypertension.
	Blood cholesterol.
Dewey Number:	616.13206

International distribution by Pineapple Media Ltd (www.pineapple-media.com)
Cover photographs: Rod Stewart
Design: Jo Hunt
Photos and illustrations by agreement with international agencies, photographers and illustrators from Thinkstock.
Printed in China

Why this book matters

Walk around a 'heart' ward in any hospital around the world and you'll see men and women of all shapes, sizes and ages. But the vast majority have something in common – they had lived with at least one risk factor associated with coronary heart disease in the lead-up to their hospital stay. Most alarming, though, is that most of these risk factors are easily reversible and in many cases preventable.

The global statistics around coronary heart disease, heart attack and stroke are truly alarming. And as for the rates of high blood pressure and cholesterol, both major risk factors of the above conditions, well they too are extraordinary. The tragedy is that the rates are rising worldwide, despite how easy it can be in many circumstances to reduce risk.

In this book, we'll take a good look at what high blood pressure and high cholesterol are and why they can be so dangerous, and, in particular, why atherosclerosis, or plaque build-up in the arteries, is the most significant consequence of these conditions and causal factor of heart attack, stroke and coronary heart disease. We'll look at the risk factors associated with high blood pressure and cholesterol and how we need to consider our overall and absolute risks when determining how we manage them. Surprising to many is that often it's possible to treat high readings without pharmacological intervention. Finally, we'll look at ways we can reduce or reverse our risk of high blood pressure and high cholesterol, and, ultimately, our risk of heart attack, stroke and coronary heart disease. And perhaps we might even learn a few tips that could help us to avoid a stay on the heart ward of our city's hospital.

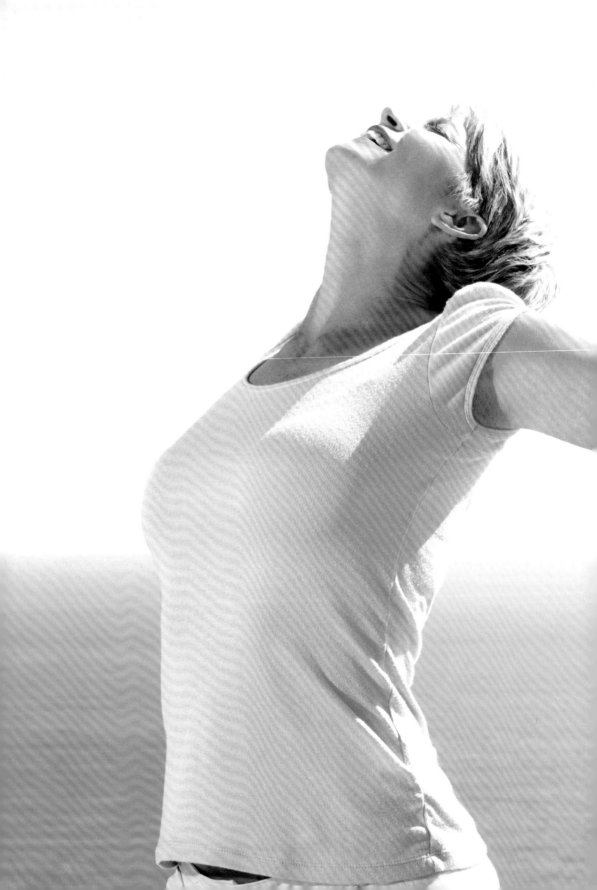

Contents

Introduction

As a journalist, I always loved writing health-related feature stories and interviewing the courageous people who had overcome some pretty horrific health issues. But as much as I empathised with them and admired their strength, I didn't rush out to buy a gym membership, nor hire a personal trainer/chef/life-coach to help me improve my life expectancy.

That wake-up call arrived when I started work at one of Melbourne's largest hospitals. I worked in the Public Relations Department, and would do 'ward rounds', trying to find good news stories to pitch to the media. Walking around the 'heart' ward, I was struck by how random the patients were. There were men and women of all shapes, sizes and ages. I learnt that the vast majority of these patients had lived with the risk factors associated with coronary heart disease in the lead-up to their hospital stay. Most alarming however, was that most of these risk factors were easily reversible and in many cases preventable. I realised that I could probably tick the box for a few of those risk factors, and it could quite easily have been me lying in that hospital bed.

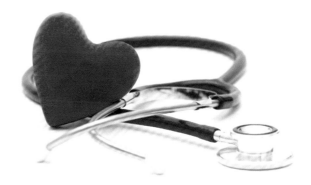

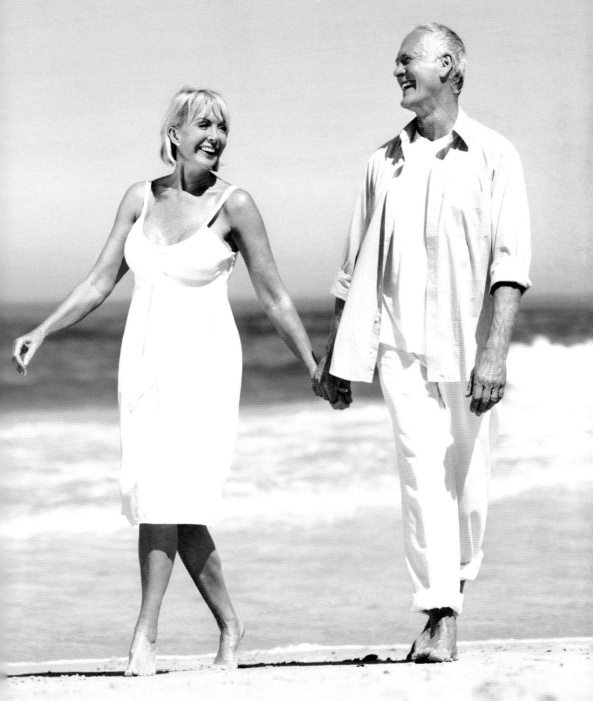

We'll look at ways we can reduce or reverse our risk of high blood pressure and high cholesterol, and, ultimately, our risk of heart attack, stroke and coronary heart disease.

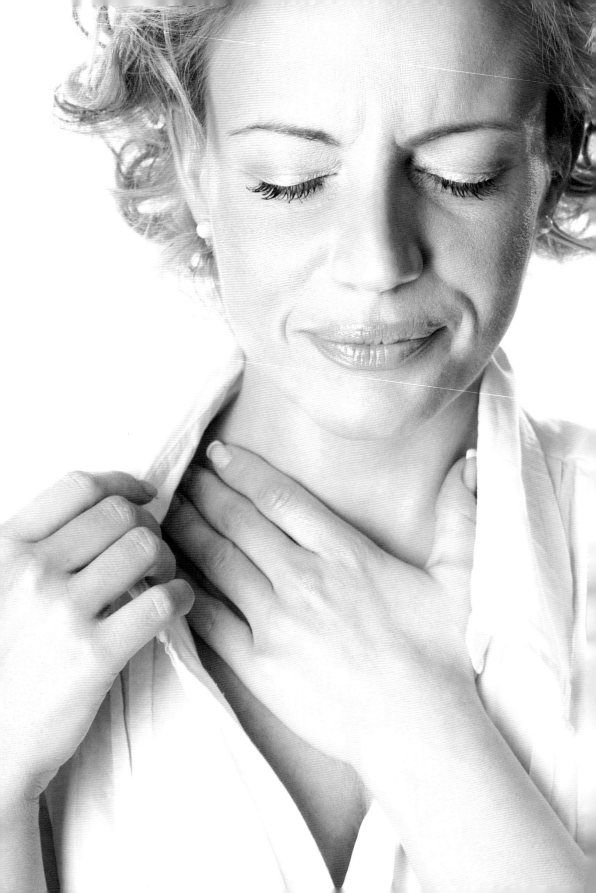

Understanding high blood pressure

What is High Blood Pressure?

High blood pressure, or hypertension, is one of the major risk factors for heart attack and stroke. Particularly when paired with other risk factors, the condition can be devastating. It's not a problem isolated to the western world. It's a global issue, and, despite being preventable, easily detected and easily treated, it's on the rise. 1.6 billion people worldwide are expected to have the condition by 2025.

So many of us have heard about hypertension – 'Granddad's blood pressure was through the roof'; 'My wife's blood pressure was high when she was pregnant'; 'Uncle Eddie was on blood pressure tablets for 40 years' – but what exactly is it?

Basically, hypertension means that your blood pressure is consistently higher than the recommended level. Any novice pub-quizzer or high school student could probably tell you that the 'ideal' blood pressure reading is 120/80 (said as '120 over 80'). But understanding just what those figures actually mean, well, the answer to that question is not as widely known (and go straight to the top of the class if you know what the instrument that measures blood pressure is called!) To put it very simply, a blood pressure reading is similar to the concept of air pressure in a car tyre. It measures the force pushing outwards on your arterial walls – the physical pressure inside the blood vessels.

Measured in units known as millimetres of mercury (mmHg), the top reading is the systolic pressure, which is the pressure in the arteries when the heart beats and pumps blood through your arteries. The bottom reading is the diastolic pressure, and measures the pressure in the arteries when the heart is relaxing between beats.

While 120/80mmHg is commonly accepted as the ideal blood pressure reading, unless a doctor has told you otherwise, your blood pressure should sit below 140/90mmHg. For those with heart or circulatory disease, or if you have diabetes or kidney disease, your blood pressure should measure below 130/80mmHg.

Diagnostic levels of blood pressure

Grade	Systolic (mmHg)	Diastolic (mmHg)
Normal	Less than 120	Less than 80
High normal	120 – 139	80 – 89
Mild hypertension	140 – 159	90 – 99
Moderate hypertension	160 – 179	100 – 109
Severe hypertension	Greater than or equal to 180	Greater than or equal to 110

How do you know if your blood pressure is high?

One of the major reasons why hypertension is so prevalent in the community is because high blood pressure is not usually something you can feel or notice. If you don't have your blood pressure tested, then you may not know that you're one of the millions of people worldwide going about your daily life unaware of your increased risk of permanently damaging your heart, brain, eyes and kidneys. You may not know that heart attack, heart failure, stroke and kidney failure are very real dangers.

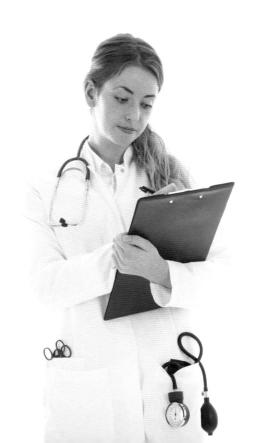

How do you test for high blood pressure?

Most of us have seen the instrument used to measure blood pressure, either on one of the many television hospital dramas, in our kids' dress-up doctor's bag or, most likely, in our GP's rooms. The instrument is called a sphygmomanometer. The painless technique involves the use of an inflatable cuff that is wrapped around the upper arm. The cuff is then inflated until the blood flow through the arm's arteries is cut off. The cuff is then slowly deflated and a stethoscope is used to hear the sound of the blood flow resuming and disappearing. The pressure at which sounds start is the systolic pressure, the maximum pressure developed by the beating heart, and the lowest pressure between heartbeats – the diastolic pressure – is recorded when sound disappears.

While resting blood pressure is generally considered normal when it's below 140/90mmHg, blood pressure can, in fact, be variable. This is why doctors tend not to treat blood pressure based on a one-off elevated reading.

Did you know

'If you know that a sphygmomanometer is the cuffed instrument used to measure blood pressure then it might be time to submit an application for *Who Wants to be a Millionaire*.'

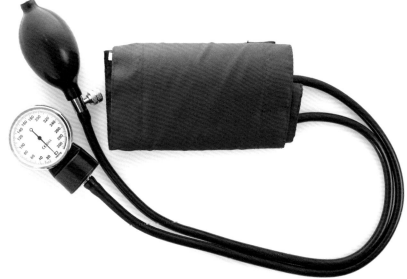

What can cause blood pressure to vary?

There are a multitude of reasons why blood pressure can fluctuate. Blood pressure can be elevated transiently by factors including recent physical activity, caffeine consumption, smoking, your emotional state, stress and even some things as benign as talking. In fact, just seeing your GP approaching with the sphygmomanometer can be enough to trigger a blood pressure elevation, which is why hypertension is not diagnosed until resting blood pressure is consistently elevated over several visits to your doctor. While there are automated blood pressure machines available for home use, it is vital that the equipment is reliable and validated to ensure an accurate picture is drawn. So having a professional measure your blood pressure is probably the best way to gain an accurate picture.

In some cases, patients can be fitted with ambulatory monitors over a 24-hour period to gather more comprehensive blood pressure measures. This type of testing can be particularly helpful as it reads the patient's blood pressure during normal activities, which can help with a more conclusive diagnosis of hypertension.

But why are these readings significant? The idea of comparing blood pressure to that of a car tyre offers a simplistic explanation to this vitally important bodily function. Further explanation reveals just how critical good blood pressure is to our health. Blood pressure is the driving force for blood to travel around the body in order to deliver freshly oxygenated and nutrient-rich blood to the organs. So, to help fully understand what blood pressure is, to learn how important it is to maintain a healthy reading, and what the consequences of poor heart health can be, it firstly helps to understand how our heart works.

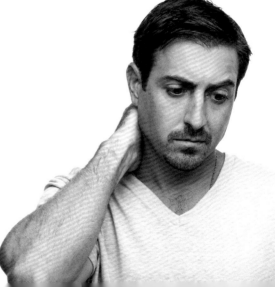

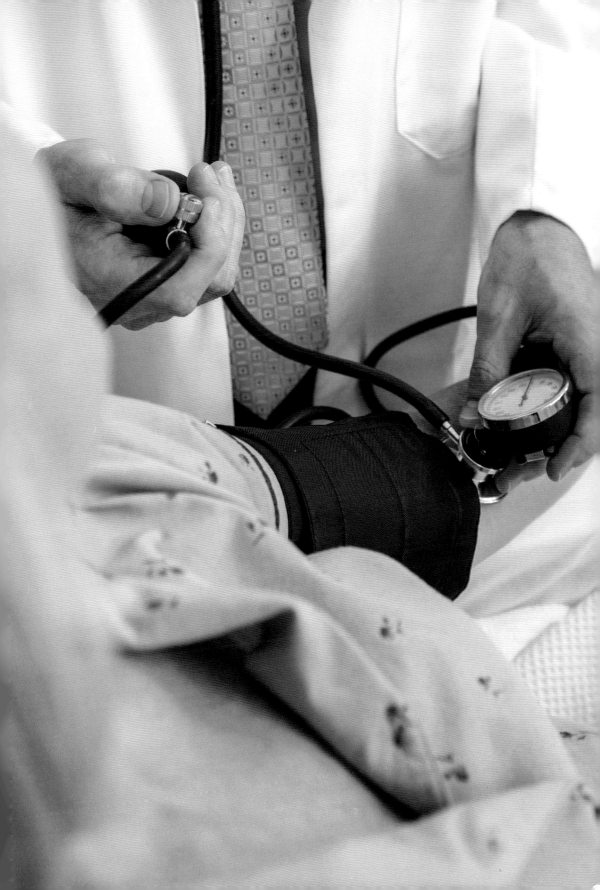

How the heart works

The heart is a clenched fist-sized muscle found behind, and slightly to the left, of the breastbone. It acts like the body's pump – pumping blood around to the body's organs and beating about 100,000 times per day.

A wall separates the left side of the heart from the right side to protect oxygen-rich blood from mixing with oxygen-poor blood, and each side has two chambers – one large and one small. The small chambers are called the right and left atrium, while the large chambers are the heart's pumping chambers and called the left and right ventricle. There are also four valves within the heart, each tasked with ensuring blood moves in the right direction. They open and close once every heartbeat, in one direction and, like the opening of a gate, will only open when pushed on.

The right side of the heart is the 'collecting side'. It collects the blood that is returning from the rest of the body. The blood that is collected here is low in oxygen – sometimes referred to as blue blood – as the oxygen and nutrients that were present in the circulating blood have already been delivered to the body's organs and tissues.

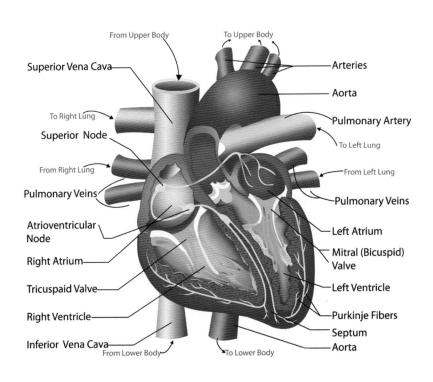

From Upper Body — To Upper Body

Superior Vena Cava — Arteries

Aorta

To Right Lung — Pulmonary Artery

Superior Node — To Left Lung

From Right Lung — From Left Lung

Pulmonary Veins — Pulmonary Veins

Atrioventricular Node — Left Atrium

Right Atrium — Mitral (Bicuspid) Valve

Tricuspaid Valve — Left Ventricle

Right Ventricle — Purkinje Fibers

Septum

Inferior Vena Cava — Aorta

From Lower Body — To Lower Body

The oxygen-poor blood passes through the right atrium into the right ventricle, which pumps the blood through the pulmonary artery to the lungs, where the blood is refreshed with a new supply of oxygen. This oxygen-rich blood is red in colour and enters the left side of the heart via the pulmonary vein. It is then pushed into the left ventricle, which pumps this oxygenated blood through the aorta then around to the rest of the body to supply tissues with oxygen.

This pumping action, which pushes the blood between the chambers and around the body to where it's needed is, in effect, your heart beating. A beating heart contracts - called systole - and relaxes – called diastole (remember your blood pressure reading contains systolic and diastolic measurements). During systole, your ventricles contract, forcing blood into the vessels that carry blood to the lungs and body, like the squeezing of a tomato sauce bottle. When the ventricles relax during diastole, they fill with blood from the upper chambers - the atria - and then the beating heart cycle begins again.

Like every other organ, the heart also needs blood for nourishment. It too has a supply of blood vessels, called coronary arteries, which extend over the surface of the heart and then branch into smaller capillaries.

The heart also has electrical wiring, which keeps the heart beating in a coordinated rhythm by delivering a signal to pump. This 'normal' rhythm keeps our blood circulating. It's this continuous cycle of exchanging oxygen-poor blood with oxygen-rich blood that keeps us alive.

So, we know that for our very survival, we need our heart to beat so it can pump oxygenated blood around our body. When there's interference with this process, that's when things start to go wrong – sometimes terminally.

Why is hypertension problematic?

There are so many reasons why hypertension is dangerous – heart attack, stroke, aneurysms, tissue damage and organ failure. And over time, if it's not treated, your heart may become enlarged, which makes your heart pump less effectively, and heart failure could occur.

But if you think back to our tyre example, if we apply too much force then serious problems arise. So, we make sure we don't over-inflate our tyres as we don't want to weaken them, and we certainly don't want to pump them up so much that they pop. And the same applies to our arteries. Healthy arteries are made of muscle and a semi-flexible tissue so they can stretch as blood pumps through them. When you're hypertensive, blood is pumped more forcefully through the arteries, so they have to stretch more to allow blood to flow easily through them. If the force of the blood flow is regularly high, the flexible tissue that makes up the arteries' walls can stretch beyond its healthy limit. This can cause a multitude of problems.

Firstly, this overstretching can create vascular weaknesses – weaknesses in the blood vessels. The weaknesses make the blood vessels susceptible to rupture. These ruptures cause strokes and aneurysms.

A second issue is vascular scarring. The overstretching can cause microscopic tears in the blood vessels that can leave scar tissue on the arteries' and veins' walls. This is problematic because the scar tissue and little rips act like nets and can catch debris including cholesterol, plaque or blood cells as they travel through the vessels. Trapped blood cells can then form blood clots that may narrow or even block the arteries. Sometimes, the clots can break away and then travel through the bloodstream blocking the vessels where the clot is too large to continue on its path. This can result in the blood supply being cut off to the parts of the body on the other side of the blockage that are reliant on the blood flow. Heart attacks or strokes are often the result of a blood clot blockage.

Similarly, and most significantly in understanding the dangers of high blood pressure, and for that matter cholesterol, the cholesterol and plaque build-up from the scar tissue 'net' that catches this passing debris can cause the blood supply to be restricted or cut off on the other side of the blockage. This build-up in the arterial walls is called atherosclerosis and is the major issue with raised blood pressure. With some arteries blocked, the heart is forced to work harder to service the body because there is increased pressure on the rest of the system. Furthermore, pieces of plaque could break off and travel elsewhere around the body and block vessels completely. The results could be catastrophic – heart attack or stroke.

If tissue is not supplied with oxygenated blood, the tissue may become damaged or even die. When blockages occur, the tissue on the other side of the blockage doesn't receive enough of this oxygen-rich blood so it's easy to see how tissues and organs can fail if you are hypertensive.

Furthermore, the circulatory system has to work harder when arteries are blocked and not functioning at capacity. The American Heart Association likens this increased workload to a home's plumbing: 'Think of it this way: In a home where several faucets [taps] are open and running, the water pressure flowing out of any one faucet is lower. But when pipes get clogged and therefore narrow, the pressure is much greater. And if all the household water is flowing through only one faucet, the pressure is higher still.'

Heart failure is a very real risk when arteries lose their elasticity from the build-up of cholesterol and plaque or tissue scarring. The heart has to pump harder to get blood into the arteries, which can result in damage to the heart's muscles and valves, and heart failure can result.

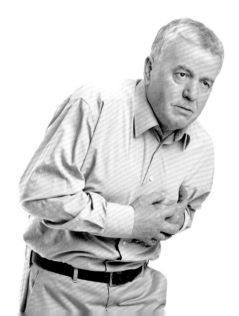

Differences between heart attack, cardiac arrest, stroke and heart failure

There is often confusion between these terms so here's a basic description of each.

Heart attack

A heart attack occurs when the flow of oxygen-rich blood to a section of the heart muscle is cut-off, stopping the supply of oxygen to that section of the heart. If the blood supply isn't restored quickly, the part of the heart muscle with no supply starts to die.

The most common cause of heart attacks is coronary heart disease, which is a condition whereby fatty materials, called plaque, build up inside the coronary arteries (the pipes that supply blood to the heart). This build-up in the arteries is called atherosclerosis. If an area of plaque cracks, other materials found in blood, including cholesterol, stick to the damaged area and form blood clots. It is these blood clots that create blockages in the coronary arteries, which in turn lead to heart attacks.

Cardiac Arrest

A cardiac arrest occurs when your heart stops pumping blood around the body. It is caused when the heart's electrical system malfunctions. If you have a cardiac arrest, you lose consciousness almost at once. There are also no other signs of life such as breathing or movement. While a heart attack may cause cardiac arrest and sudden death, the terms don't mean the same thing.

Source: British Heart Foundation

Heart Failure

Heart failure is a chronic, progressive condition in which the heart muscle is unable to pump enough blood through to meet the body's need for blood and oxygen. Basically, the heart can't keep up with its workload. At first, the heart tries to make up for this by:

Enlarging When the heart chamber enlarges, it stretches more and can contract more strongly, so it pumps more blood.

Developing more muscle mass The increase in muscle mass occurs because the contracting cells of the heart get bigger. This lets the heart pump more strongly, at least initially.

Pumping faster This helps to increase the heart's output.

The body also tries to compensate in other ways: The blood vessels narrow to keep blood pressure up, trying to make up for the heart's loss of power.

The body diverts blood away from less important tissues and organs to maintain flow to the most vital organs – the heart and brain.

Source: American Heart Association

Stroke

Stroke is a disease that affects the arteries leading to and within the brain. A stroke occurs when a blood vessel that carries oxygen and nutrients to the brain is either blocked by a clot or bursts (ruptures). When that happens, part of the brain cannot get the blood and oxygen it needs, so it and brain cells die.

Source: American Stroke Association

Other health consequences

While high blood pressure is most often mentioned in the same breath as heart attack, heart failure and stroke, hypertension can also be responsible for a number of other health complications.

Loss of vision

The blood vessels in the eyes can become strained when you have high blood pressure. The vessels may narrow or bleed when they are exposed to too much blood pressure force and the optic nerve may also swell, reducing the ability to see well.

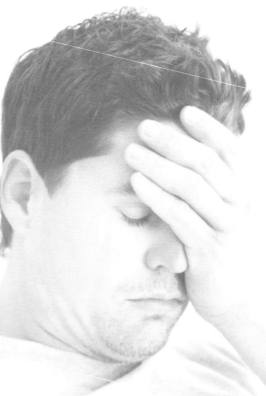

Kidney damage

Our kidneys are densely packed with arteries to accommodate the high volume of blood that flows through them. High blood pressure can cause a narrowing, weakening or even hardening of the kidneys' arteries. This damage means the kidney tissue doesn't receive enough blood. As a result, the kidneys lose their ability to filter blood and regulate the fluid, hormones, acids and salts in the body. And in a double-blow, healthy kidneys are also responsible for producing a hormone that helps the body to regulate blood pressure. When kidneys are damaged, this production process is affected so the kidneys fail to regulate blood pressure as they should. The kidneys eventually fail as more and more arteries are blocked.

Erectile Dysfunction

In order to achieve and sustain an erection, the penis needs effective blood flow through the veins and arteries. As we've already learned, high blood pressure can reduce or cut off blood flow, therefore sufficient blood flow to the penis may be compromised if a man is hypertensive. The arterial system is at the heart of a number of medical-related erectile dysfunction issues.

What are the causes of high blood pressure?

Unfortunately, there isn't always a categorical explanation for the cause of high blood pressure. In fact, only 5-10 per cent of people with high blood pressure can say with certainty that they know why they are hypertensive. This type of high blood pressure is called secondary hypertension because it is caused by a pre-existing problem. Some of these explanations include hormonal imbalances and kidney diseases that result from genetic complaints, a structural abnormality of the aorta, tumours, and narrowing of certain arteries. More often than not, if the original condition is corrected, the secondary hypertension is also corrected. For the other 90-95 per cent of people with hypertension, they are said to have essential hypertension. With no precise medical explanation, these cases are likely to be the result of a number of environmental/lifestyle factors and genetic factors that work together to raise blood pressure. We'll explore the risk factors associated with blood pressure in-depth in a later chapter. But briefly, they are:

- Family history
- Advancing age
- Gender
- Lack of physical activity
- Overweight and obesity
- Too much salt in your diet
- Regularly drinking too much alcohol

There is also some connection between the following factors and high blood pressure:

- Smoking
- Stress
- Sleep apnoea

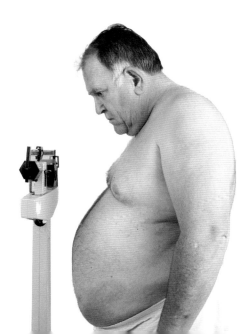

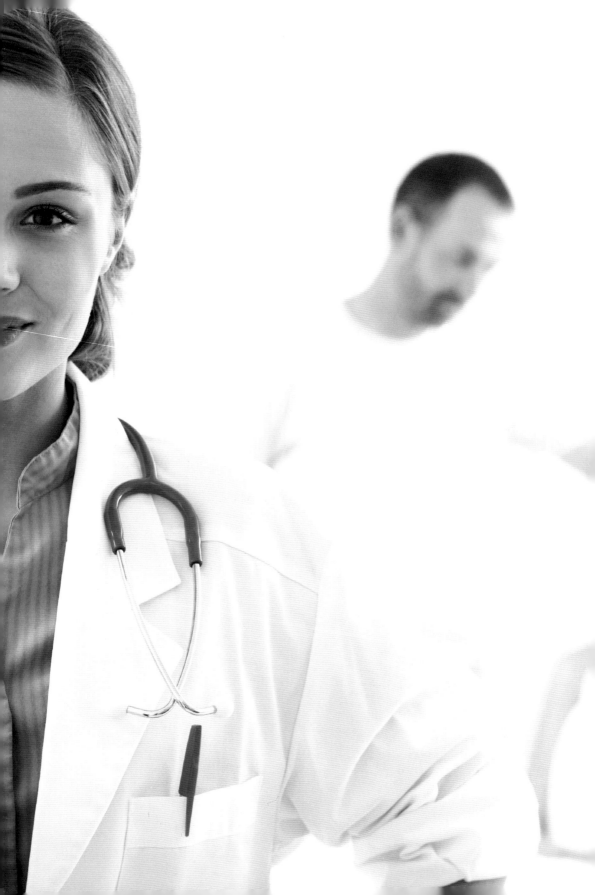

Understanding high cholesterol

The mere mention of the word cholesterol is often enough to send you bolting to the fridge to throw out the dozen eggs you bought yesterday (I wonder if I can consider that flurry of activity as my doctor-prescribed exercise for the day!). But cholesterol itself isn't actually bad. It's essential for many of the body's metabolic processes. It's a type of fat, is a part of all animal cells and our body is really good at making its own, so we don't need to help it along by eating foods high in cholesterol.

Cholesterol – a white, insoluble, waxy substance – is produced by the liver, as well as most cells in the body. It travels around in our blood, carried by lipoproteins – think of these as little couriers – to where our body needs it. We need a small amount of blood cholesterol because the body uses it to build the structure of cell membranes, to make hormones (including oestrogen, testosterone and adrenal hormones), to help your metabolism work efficiently (for example, cholesterol is essential for your body to produce vitamin D) and to produce bile acids (which helps to digest fat and absorb important nutrients).

So, because cholesterol can't dissolve in the blood, it moves around the body by two key transport systems – low-density lipoprotein (LDL) and high-density lipoprotein (HDL). These two types of lipids, along with triglycerides and Lp(a) cholesterol, make up your total cholesterol count, which can be determined through a blood test. It's LDL which carries most of the cholesterol that's delivered to cells. It's often called 'bad' cholesterol because when too much LDL circulates in the blood, reaching high levels in the bloodstream, it can slowly build up in the inner walls of the arteries feeding the heart and brain. Together with other substances, it can form plaque - a thick, hard deposit that can narrow the arteries and make them less

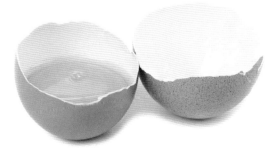

flexible. This condition is called atherosclerosis and, as with raised blood pressure, is probably the biggest issue around this condition. If a clot forms and subsequently blocks a narrowed artery, heart attack or stroke can result.

On the other hand, HDL is referred to as 'good' cholesterol. About one-quarter to one-third of blood cholesterol is carried by HDL. It's considered to be the good cholesterol because it helps to remove excess cholesterol out of the cells, including the arteries' cells, thus protecting against heart attack. It helps coat the arteries like a protective oil, helping to prevent blockages and carries cholesterol away from the arteries and back to the liver, where it's passed from the body. Therefore, low levels of HDL (less than 40mg/dL for men and less than 50mg/dL for women) also increase the risk of heart disease.

Triglyceride is also a form of fat that the body produces. Elevated levels of triglyceride can be due to obesity/overweight, physical inactivity, smoking, excess alcohol consumption, and a high carbohydrate diet (60 per cent or more of total daily kilojoules). Those with high triglyceride levels often have a high total cholesterol count that includes high LDL and low HDL levels. Many people with heart disease or diabetes also seem to have high levels of this form of fat.

Lp(a) cholesterol is a genetic variation of LDL and a major risk factor for the premature development of fatty arterial deposits. While little is known about Lp(a), it is thought that it may interact with substances found in artery walls and contributes to the build-up of fatty deposits.

How are cholesterol levels tested?

A doctor can determine your fasting lipoprotein profile by performing a blood test after a fasting period of nine to twelve hours. The test gives information about your total cholesterol, your LDL, HDL and triglyceride levels. In America, the levels are measured in milligrams per decilitre of blood (mg/dL), while in the United Kingdom and Australia, cholesterol is measured in units called millimols per litre (mmol/l) of blood. They provide useful information for your doctor to determine your heart disease risk in conjunction with your other risk factors, a topic that will be discussed at length later. The American Heart Association recommends all people over the age of twenty should have a fasting lipoprotein profile every five years.

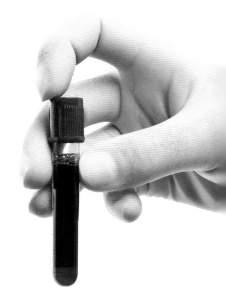

Understanding cholesterol test results

While a total cholesterol level reading gives a broad idea of where your cholesterol's at, breaking it down is more useful. Health authorities' recommended levels vary from one country to the next but there is consensus that with HDL, the higher the reading, the better. The American Heart Association considers 60mg/dL of HDL as being protective against heart disease. Less than 40mg/dL of HDL is considered a low reading for men and a major risk factor for heart disease, while for women, 50mg/dL is considered to be low. The UK recommendation is for HDL levels to be above 1mmol/l.

In contrast, the lower your LDL level, the better and the lower your risk of heart attack and stroke. Less than 100mg/dL is considered to be the optimal LDL concentration in the US, while 130-159mg/dL is borderline high, and anything greater is considered high. The UK suggests you should aim to have an LDL of less than 2mmol/l. But authorities worldwide agree that these readings should not be used in isolation to determine what course of action, if any, is required. A healthy level for you may not be healthy for someone else, so you should discuss your results with your doctor to work out the best plan for you and what is considered a safe concentration of each blood lipid.

People who have high triglyceride levels generally do so because of their lifestyle habits, however, there are underlying diseases or genetic disorders that can increase levels. Normal triglyceride levels vary by age and sex but less than 100mg/dL is considered to be the optimal level. A reading between 150 and 199mg/dL is borderline high, while anything above 200mg/dL is high according to the American Heart Association. In the UK, your triglyceride level should sit below 1.7mmol/l.

High cholesterol – Hypercholesterolaemia

Hypercholesterolaemia is the condition of having too much cholesterol in the blood. Every day, we produce a certain amount of cholesterol. Hypercholesterolaemia occurs when our system has excess cholesterol because of either a genetic factor or our diet.

Not unlike high blood pressure (hypertension), there are no symptoms of hypercholesterolaemia. The only way to know you have a problem is to have a blood test.

Why does high cholesterol matter?

Atherosclerosis is the major reason why high cholesterol matters. This build-up of plaque within the arteries can lead to blockages, which can cause heart attack, stroke and coronary heart disease - each of which can have deadly consequences. As your blood cholesterol rises, so does your risk of coronary heart disease. If there are also other risk factors present, the risk multiplies. Understanding your risk is therefore imperative.

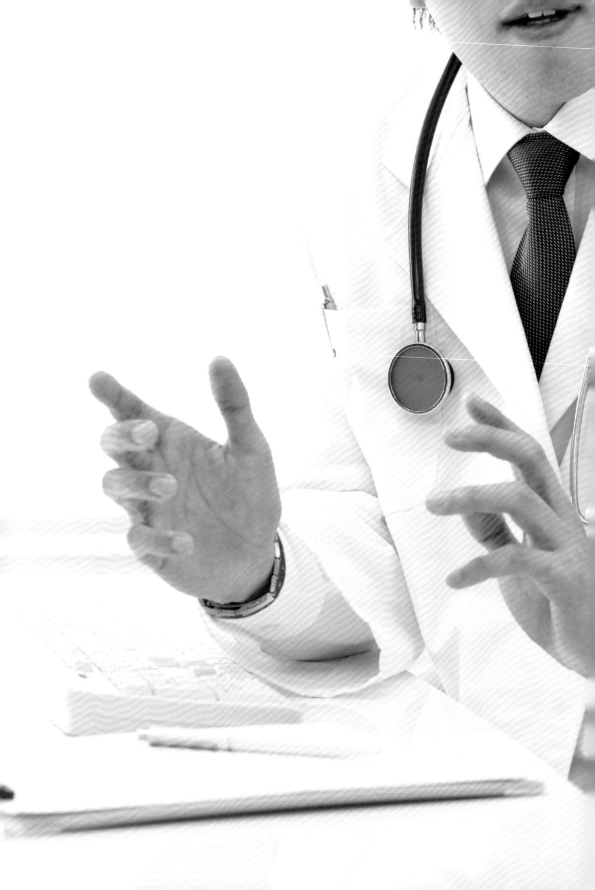

Know your risk

So far, we've looked at what high blood pressure and high cholesterol are and why they can be problematic. They can indeed have a devastating impact, but it doesn't always have to be the case. Hearing that you have mildly-elevated blood pressure or that your latest cholesterol test revealed you had a reading of 5.9mmols/l might, in fact, not be cause for major concern if these problems exist in isolation.

I recently had the opportunity to sit down with internationally-renowned interventional cardiologist Professor Ian Meredith, Director of MonashHeart in Australia and Board Member of the Australian Heart Foundation (Victorian branch). Every day, Professor Meredith sees first-hand the consequences of hypertension and hypercholesterolaemia in his hospital beds and on his catheterisation lab tables. However he also sees patients for whom he can deliver the good news that their moderately raised blood pressure reading, or their slightly elevated cholesterol, is not necessarily a condition that requires medical intervention.

For Professor Meredith, establishing the context that risks exist in is important when deciding on a treatment plan. He also believes that you should work out your absolute and overall risks of a cardiovascular event to determine the best course of action for you. I put a few questions to Professor Meredith so he could help us to understand this concept, and in his inimitable style, here's how he explained it.

If someone has a cholesterol test and their levels are a little too high, should they start taking cholesterol-lowering medication?

Let's take someone with moderately-elevated cholesterol. With cholesterol, what you have to understand is that it's just one of a series of soldiers that you might be fighting. If you're up against one single soldier, you may be able to handle him quite easily. Let's say you lived in a castle and there's one lone warrior at the castle gate called Cholesterol. He's an easy management task and may not need the help of medication to remedy but if he's actually lined up with a thousand men called Diabetes or fifty men called High Blood Pressure (or indeed both), or even half a million men called Smoking, that warrior called Cholesterol is a completely different prospect. So managing him is much harder.

So what I'm saying is, when you look at your cholesterol and how you have to manage it, you must look at it in context of who else is trying to storm the gates of your castle. If it's just one guy, you might just have to drop a boulder from the castle's parapet on his head and he's gone. But if you look out and see thousands and thousands of armed soldiers, you've got a serious battle on your hands, and therefore, you have to treat it aggressively. If you've got mildly-elevated cholesterol, in the context of no other risk factors, that's a very different prospect to mildly-elevated cholesterol in the context of other significant risk factors. So you firstly have to determine your absolute or overall risk.'

So would you only treat cholesterol if there are other risk factors for coronary heart disease? Factors like family history, smoking, lack of exercise, poor diet, diabetes and obesity?

It's true to say that there's very little benefit from treating mildly-elevated cholesterol in the absence of other significant risks in a young person who doesn't manifest heart disease. That's one warrior at the gates of the castle. He's easily dispatched, often by diet modification. But if he's there with Smoking and Diabetes, two very malignant partners, this is a very different game. Then you need to treat him with contempt and you have to bring in your big weapons.

The most important thing for people to understand is their overall burden of risks. Who else is at the gates trying to storm the castle and how big is that army against you? Then you take actions in accordance with the size of the army mounting against you. If you wind up with three opponents to fight versus one, then you take a completely different approach.'

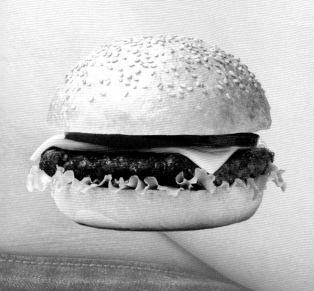

Does the same apply for people with mildly-elevated blood pressure?

That's right, the same thing applies with blood pressure. If you're a forty-year-old woman and you're otherwise well, fit and lean, exercise regularly and have mild or moderately-elevated blood pressure, then non-pharmacological approaches might be the most appropriate course of action in the first instance. If, however, you're a diabetic, then that's a very nasty ally you've got with your blood pressure, and we're now going to treat your blood pressure very differently to that of a 40-year-old woman with the same blood pressure numerical values but who is otherwise a fit and healthy person. How we treat you depends on who you line up against. The only time this rule doesn't apply is when diabetes is present. Diabetes is bad on its own. And smoking is bad on its own, but with cholesterol and blood pressure, it depends who your mates are.

I believe that you ask patients about their family history when you're weighing up treatment options. How important are genetics for patients who present with high cholesterol or blood pressure?

If dad died at 40, and dad's dad died at 40, and dad's cholesterol was mildly elevated, you'd then take a look at cholesterol in more detail. If you have severe hypercholesterolemia (severe high blood cholesterol) and you have a family history of heart disease, of course you'd treat that. It's important to ask the question. When people come along to see me with a mildly-elevated cholesterol, I'd ask, are you a diabetic, do you have high blood pressure, are you overweight, are you a smoker and did your parents die young? If the answer to those questions is yes, of course you're going to treat that mild cholesterol problem very aggressively. However if the answer to all those questions is no, then you might say, 'let's try exercise first and then we'll see how your cholesterol goes'. You've got to explain to people that the treatment recommended correlates to their level of risk.

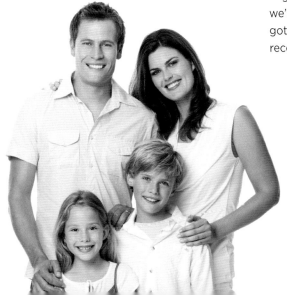

When assessing risk, you've clarified that looking at the big picture is imperative, but is it sometimes necessary to delve a little deeper for someone with high cholesterol?

One of the other major things you have to understand about cholesterol is, when making decisions to treat, not only do you look at overall risk – who else is at the gates – you then have to ask who's in that family of cholesterol? The total concentration reading doesn't tell you necessarily the make-up of the family. We look first at the total concentration, because more is bad generally unless you've got a high HDL, and that's how we screen the population. So, when you measure cholesterol in plasma, it's a family and not one single molecule. It's like all families, there are some troublesome ones and there are good ones. There are model citizens that might go on to be the Prime Minister or state governor and then there are the really bad ones who may end up in prison. Cholesterol is a whole family of molecules. There are atherogenic ones, LDL, IDL, VLDL, that contribute to build up in the arteries, and there are less atherogenic, sometimes helpful ones, like HDL. So you have to look at what proportion of your cholesterol profile is good. This is because you often see people who are referred for cholesterol management and their cholesterol reading is six, and then you find out that they have a HDL of two. Well if you have a HDL of two, you're about as likely to have heart disease as being kicked to death by a duck. Unless there's a significant family history or some rare malignant HDL syndrome, the likelihood of you having heart disease is low and you're probably going to do well.

These are, of course, generalisations, but they're reasonably strong generalisations. You can have malignant HDL, a condition where you have loads of HDL but it's all corrupt, like a bad police force, but that's pretty rare. Mostly, if you have a big police force, the town is pretty safe and not much happens. If you have a low level of HDL, and even a modest elevation of LDL, that's far more problematic than a moderately severe elevation of LDL in a context of normal HDL.

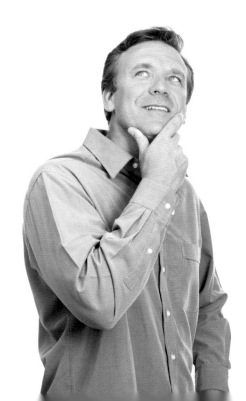

So what are the steps that health practitioners take when deciding how to treat a patient with raised cholesterol or blood pressure?

The two things you look at are the milieu of risk factors for the patient – you'd never treat cholesterol medically without knowing the milieu (who's at the gate trying to knock the door down). If he's out on his own, we might just leave him out there making a noise, perhaps not even bothering to deal with him because he's not going to harm anything. Then if you're a little bit worried, you'd look at the second thing, the family of cholesterol, and ask how many good ones are in the family and how many bad ones are there. And if there are lots of good ones in the family, you might tolerate one or two of the naughty ones because overall the family's pretty good. So, that's how you deal with it.

It's critical to put things into context and it's the same with blood pressure. Take the classic 45-year-old woman who has mildly-elevated blood pressure, and she's worried because her mum had high blood pressure. So you look at them and ask yourself if they're normal weight or are they overweight, do they have diabetes, do they not have diabetes, do they smoke or do they not smoke, do they have high cholesterol? All of these factors are multiplicative not additive. The risk multiplies, they're not simply added together, so three and two is not five, it's six, and three and four is not seven, it's twelve (i.e., one risk, say high cholesterol, has a risk factor of three

and the second risk, high blood pressure, has a risk factor of four. The overall risk is not three plus four, it's three multiplied by four. Together they have a risk factor of twelve). That means cholesterol and blood pressure in combination is far worse than just having one, and that diabetes, or any other risk factor, with any of those two conditions is much, much more problematic. So in those situations, you treat each of those issues far more vigorously because they exist in tandem.

For blood pressure patients, doctors would look at them, look at the context of all the risk factors and then ask what their absolute risk of something going wrong is. If their absolute risk of something going wrong in the short term is low and there's no family history of stroke or anything like that, then you'd suggest perhaps managing that issue by reducing salt in your diet, reducing your alcohol, taking regular exercise, and then waiting to see how you go for a while. Quite often, their blood pressure would improve.

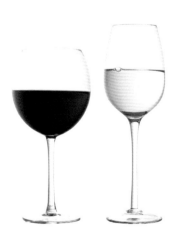

So it's pretty important then to understand what your risks are?

One of the problems with high blood pressure and cholesterol is that often you don't know you have a problem because you're usually asymptomatic. So most people don't have any idea that they've got them and therefore don't have them measured. One of the most important global campaigns in world health is knowing what your cardiovascular risks are. When I was a child, my parents didn't know their risks at all. They, and the people from their generation, only went to the doctor when they got sick and then when something went wrong they'd say, 'Oh no, I've had a heart attack, or stroke or have cancer'. There was no preventative screening whatsoever. It was just an accepted thing. That's what you did and if something went wrong that was a play of chance and unfortunately you were struck with it. Whereas these days, most people would say health is more like a bank account. I will occasionally look at the bank statements to see how much is in there and who is taking withdrawals, and you might find there are a few withdrawals that you didn't actually account for. There's a growing proportion of people who are interested in knowing their health status before things start to go wrong. And given that in the twenty-first century heart disease is going to be a major problem, one of the big things is to have people understand at a young age what their burden of risk factors are and how that's going to play throughout their life because a lot of the time, the risks are so easy to modify, with the exception of genetics – you can't change your parents. But you can do things about your cholesterol, your blood pressure, your weight, and your dietary habits.

Knowing your risk profile makes reducing your chance of heart disease a lot easier. So I'd encourage people to find out, and then once they do know their risk profile, understand what that means in absolute terms for them. When people say to you your cholesterol is high – for example you're at 20 per cent higher risk of having a stroke – you say, 'Wow, 20 per cent, that's a one-in-five greater risk of having a stroke'. However if that risk is one in five but your absolute risk of having a stroke is one in one million, what does that mean? It now means you're a one in 800,000 chance rather than one in one million. Knowing what your absolute risk of events are helps you to understand and manage that. If you're at a high absolute risk of events, of course you manage risk factors more aggressively. It's just simply looking over the castle walls and seeing a force amassing against your castle that's going to cause you big grief so you've got to clean them up. And the bigger it is, the bigger the weapons you use. People are obsessed with just numerology. They look at their numbers and say I've got to treat this, but you've got to understand context. If nobody in your family ever died of heart disease, you're incredibly fit and everything about your profile is relatively normal, then you probably don't have to do a great deal. However you might get to age sixty and then say, 'perhaps I'll do some stress testing or imaging to check that everything's in accordance with my risk'.

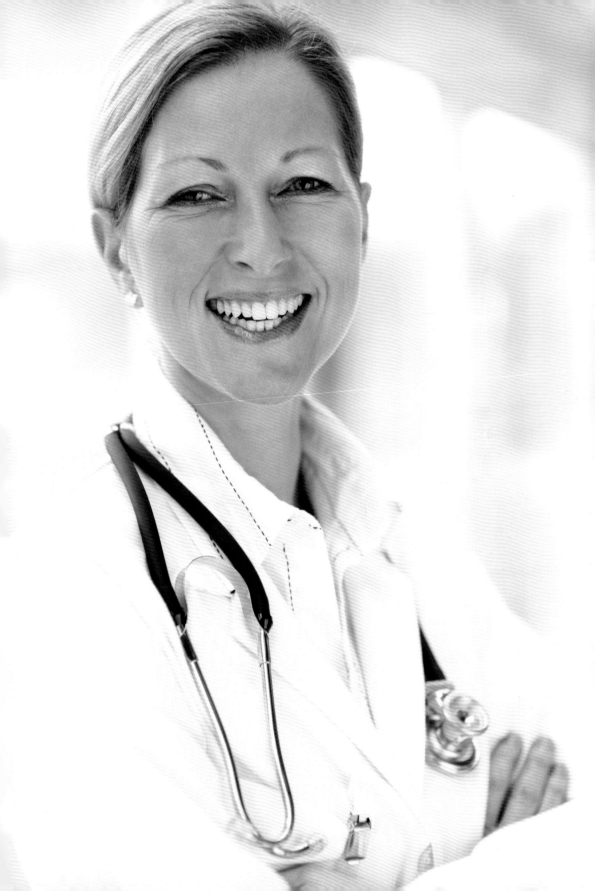

So overall risk is the taking into context all of the factors that contribute to the development of heart disease, and absolute risk is your personal risk of something going wrong?

Issues like high blood pressure or high cholesterol in isolation are merely things that lead to the development of atherosclerosis and changes to the arteries that could eventually lead to heart attack, stroke or peripheral vascular disease. Treating any one of these in isolation isn't going to help you if the others are rampantly out of control. Similarly, treating one if you don't have the others and if it's only mild might be a waste of time because your absolute risk might be so low. So, establish overall risk and then absolute risk. Overall risk is what else is in the game and then absolute risk is what your personal risk of something going wrong is. If your personal risk is incredibly low, there can be some inertia to treatment, and rightly so. This is because the chances of something going wrong with you in that respect, even though that little bit of you is wrong, is quite low. I see it all the time where people look at their cholesterol and say, 'it's 4.5 so I need to treat it'. I'd say, 'you don't have to because your personal risk is so low'. But they counter that and say they're told anything over 3.5 needs to be treated, and I retort by saying you're more likely to be struck by lightning than for that to cause you a problem. But, if you came in after a heart attack and your cholesterol is five, that's very different because you've already got a past track record - you're already a prior offender.

In summary, you're not advising people to ignore conditions like hypertension and hypercholesterolaemia if they occur in isolation or are only slightly higher than recommended? You believe they should seek the advice of a doctor to work out the best course of action for them, which in many cases may not include pharmacological intervention?

Most people who have heart disease have a little bit of everything and not a whole lot of one thing. That's my favourite saying. People diagnosed with heart disease say, 'But my cholesterol wasn't that bad', and I'd say, 'But your blood pressure wasn't that bad either; you're only a little bit diabetic, you're only a little bit overweight and you smoke five cigarettes a day, not twenty. The soldiers knocking at the gate are only five foot four not six foot two but there's a lot of them, and they're multiplicative not additive. Every risk factor multiplies your overall risk. Most people who run into trouble have a little bit of everything and not a whole lot of one thing and they get into trouble because they fly under the radar. If you had a cholesterol of 30, everybody would know about it and they'd all be treating you. But if you had a cholesterol of five and a bit, you're a little bit overweight, your blood pressure's up a little bit and you have the odd cigarette at parties at the weekend, people are not really noticing it but when you put it all together it's quite a crime.

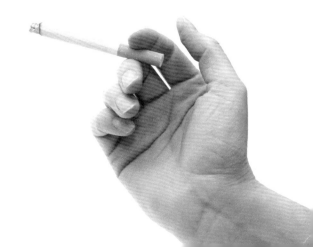

Family history is a major player when it comes to high blood pressure, Just as you inherit your eye colour from your family, you can also inherit high blood pressure.

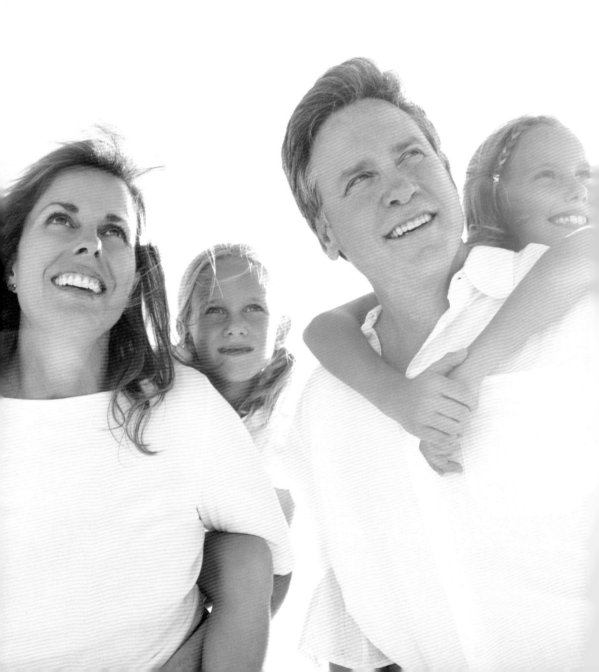

Risk factors for developing high blood pressure and high cholesterol

As Professor Meredith explained, there are numerous factors that can increase your chances of developing high blood pressure and high cholesterol. Some of them are lifestyle factors but there are others that cannot be controlled.

Family history is a major player when it comes to high blood pressure. Just as you inherit your eye and hair colour from your family, you can also inherit high blood pressure. If your parents or other close relatives have had hypertension, then you are more likely to develop the condition. And you may then pass that down to your children. Consequently,

children should also have their blood pressure checked. While you can't control your genetics, there are lifestyle choices that can be made to help you to reduce the risk associated with heredity.

As we grow older, our hypertension and cardiovascular disease risk increases. Blood vessels lose their flexibility as we age, which can increase the pressure throughout our system.

Our **gender** also affects our blood pressure risk. A higher percentage of men have hypertension that women up to the age of 45. Between the ages of 45 and 64, the percentages of men and women with high blood pressure is similar but above the age of 64, hypertension is more common in females than males.

Lack of exercise is another risk factor. Physical activity is undeniably beneficial for your heart and circulatory system. Inactivity increases not only high blood pressure but heart disease, blood vessel disease and stroke. A lack of exercise also tends to lead to **obesity/being overweight**, which is a risk factor for high blood pressure itself. The more you weigh, the more blood you need to supply oxygen and nutrients to your tissues, increasing the strain on your heart. As the volume of blood circulating through your blood vessels increases, so does the pressure on your artery walls. Excess weight can also raise blood cholesterol and triglyceride levels, and can lower good HDL cholesterol, and being obese increases your diabetes risk.

The InterHeart Study

When it comes to studies whose aims are to identify risk factors associated with heart attack, one stands out from the rest, according to Professor Meredith.

'The InterHeart Study was a study of about 25,000 people worldwide,' he says. 'When you looked across cultures there were certain things that predicted heart disease that were preserved across all cultures – when you took all other factors like socioeconomics and education etc. into account – and girth was one of them. So men with a fat belly do badly, and so do women. Initially, the findings reported that the waist-hip ratio was the factor but that's since been modified as nobody dies of a fat butt but you sure as hell get into trouble if your tummy sticks out. We now know that in helping people trying to adjust their risk profile, we try to help them improve their girth because reducing their girth and visceral fat will help to lower their overall risk.'

For most people, a waist measurement of greater than 94cm for men and 80cm for women is an indicator of internal fat deposits, which can coat the heart, kidneys, liver and pancreas and increase the risk of chronic disease.

The other risk factors for myocardial infarction (heart attack) concluded in the InterHeart Study were: abnormal lipids (high cholesterol), smoking, hypertension, diabetes, psychosocial factors, consumption of fruits, vegetables and alcohol, and regular physical activity. These factors were consistent across all ages, cultures and gender.

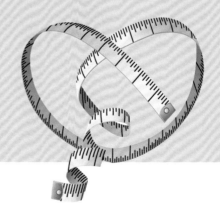

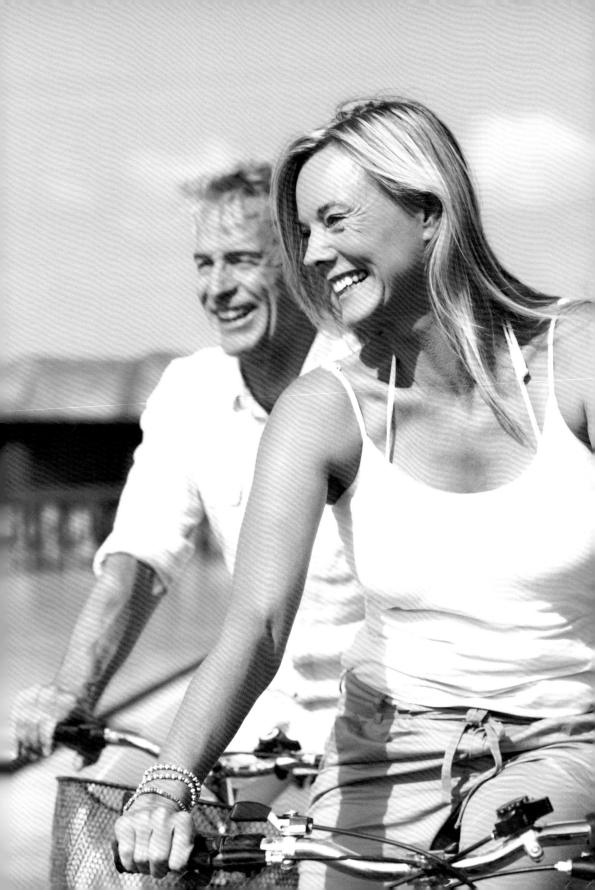

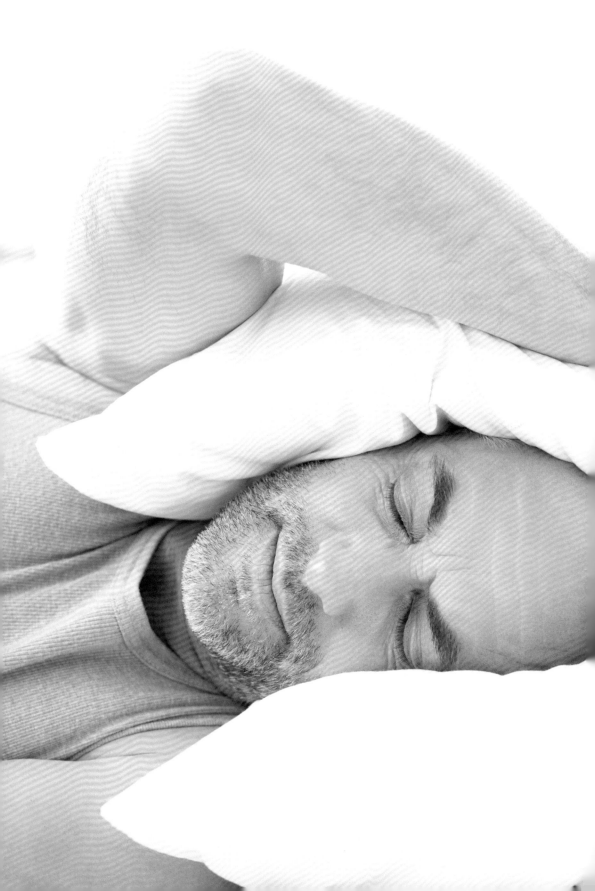

Drinking too much alcohol is another lifestyle factor that dramatically increases your risk of high blood pressure. Heart failure, stroke and irregular heartbeats are further consequences of heavy and regular use of alcohol. And the level of triglycerides in your blood is also adversely affected by excessive alcohol. Men shouldn't drink more than two standard drinks per day, while for women, it is one drink.

A poor diet, particularly one that contains too much salt, is a major risk factor for the development of high blood pressure. As already mentioned, obesity is a contributing factor for hypertension, and some people are considered 'salt-sensitive', which means that a high-salt diet raises their blood pressure. Salt is problematic because it retains excess fluid in the body which can be a burden on the heart. Potassium helps to balance the amount of sodium in your cells. So if you don't get enough potassium in your diet or retain enough potassium, you may accumulate too much sodium in your blood, which is a cause of high blood pressure. Too little vitamin D may also be a factor. It's unclear whether having too little vitamin D in your diet can lead directly to high blood pressure but it is thought that vitamin D may affect an enzyme produced by your kidneys that does affect blood pressure.

While not medically-proven, there is some connection between hypertension and stress, sleep apnoea (a life-threatening disorder in which the throat's tissues collapse and block the airway) and smoking.

Stressful situations can temporarily increase your blood pressure and while there's no scientific evidence to prove it, a relationship has been scientifically established between stress and coronary heart disease risk. Stress can contribute indirectly too. How a person deals with stress can affect your blood pressure risk. For example, people may overeat when they are stressed, fail to exercise when under pressure, or drink or smoke to relieve stress. Each of these are proven risk factors for high blood pressure.

Sleep apnoea and other chronic conditions, including high cholesterol, diabetes and kidney disease, may also increase your risk of high blood pressure. And pregnancy can also sometimes contribute to high blood pressure.

Smoking does temporarily increase blood pressure and increases your risk of damaged arteries. Exposure to second-hand smoke is also problematic. Although smoking hasn't been scientifically proven to directly cause hypertension, Professor Meredith says both smoking and hypertension cause atherosclerosis.

'Smoking increases your risk of heart attack massively,' he says. 'It accelerates atherosclerosis, the fatty deposits in your arteries, which increases your likelihood and risk of heart attack. At the end of the day, why do we treat blood pressure? Because it, and other things we treat like diabetes and high cholesterol, lead to atherosclerosis. So we treat them because they cause this atherosclerosis problem. Atherosclerosis can be manifested as a heart attack if it's in the heart, or stroke. Smoking causes heart attack and stroke directly, so it's irrelevant whether it has any bearing on blood pressure because it's taking a direct path to the problem. This guy called Smoking isn't just knocking down the door of your castle, he's parachuting himself straight in. You have to treat this enemy with incredible respect. Smoking and diaåbetes together is a terrible combination that always ends in tragedy.

What causes high cholesterol?

Like high blood pressure, there are many different factors that can contribute to high cholesterol. They include eating a diet high in saturated fats, smoking, lack of physical exercise, high alcohol intake and kidney or liver disease. And many people inherit genes from their parents or even grandparents that can cause the body to produce too much cholesterol. Having high blood pressure or diabetes also increases the risks of serious problems associated with high cholesterol.

Leading UK-based nutritional therapist Janine Fahri is treating an ever-increasing number of patients for high cholesterol from her NutriLife Clinic and her practice in Harley Street.

'The three main causes of high cholesterol are a poor diet, lack of exercise and stress. But there are other contributing factors too,' she says. 'A poor diet is one that is high in saturated fats, low in essential fats and high in refined carbohydrates, which are all the beige foods like bread, rice and pasta, as well as low in good complex carbohydrates such as oats, rye and whole grains.

'Excessive alcohol is also problematic. And we all know about smoking and what it does to you – vasodilation of the blood vessels deprives you of oxygen, prevents you from breathing and will compromise your nutrient absorption. And stress is also a factor.'

Professor Meredith says that people with a condition called dyslipidemia do not have a high cholesterol reading but what they have is dangerous.

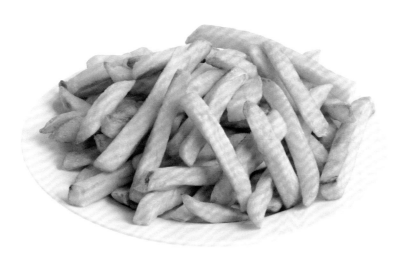

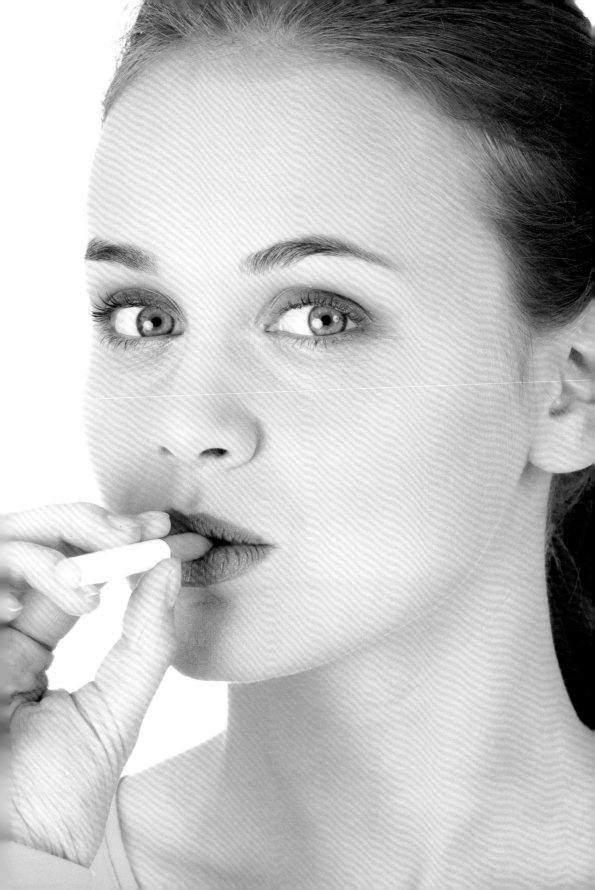

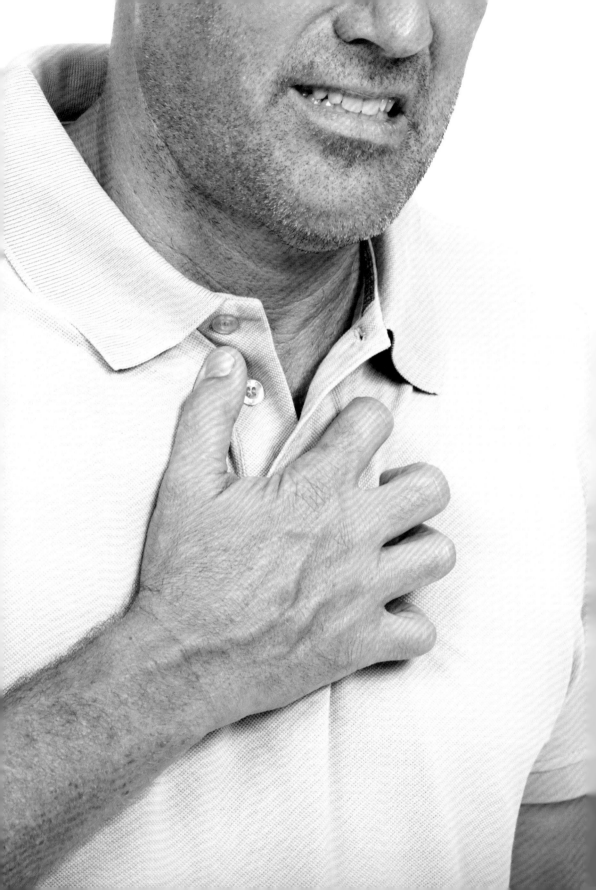

'There are lots of people who have low HDL, raised triglycerides and very small, dense LDL,' he says. 'They have what's called dyslipidemia. In people with dyslipidemia, the cholesterol level isn't high but what they have is very malignant. High triglycerides is a problem and is a marker of small, dense LDL cholesterol. Try to think of the lining of your arteries as being like carpet on the floor. Underneath the carpet is the underlay and underneath that is the floorboards. Blood vessels have three linings – carpet, underlay and floorboards. The inner line is called the intima, or endothelium, the middle one is called the media or the muscle and the outer lining is the adventitia of the fibrous capsule. If I came into your house and you've got beautiful new carpet on the floor and I threw down tennis balls, we'd be able to pick them up pretty easily. If I threw down marbles, probably a few would escape your view, but if I came in and threw sand, you'd never get it out. You'd get most of it but 50 years on it'd still be in the underlay. So, the smaller the particles, the more they have sub-intimal collection capability and hence the ability to get between the carpet and the underlay, which is really bad. So, in effect, small particles are bad. Therefore, the size of your cholesterol particles may also be an important determinant of your risk.

'What happens quite a lot is people say cholesterol levels don't matter because they had a heart attack and their cholesterol was normal. What they're really saying was that their total cholesterol number was the same as someone else who didn't have heart disease. They say that they had 4.5 millimoles per litre, and so did you, yet you didn't have heart disease. Yes, the concentration was the same, but what they don't tell you was that your family of particles were all lawyers and doctors. In their family of cholesterol particles, of the 4.5 members of the family, there were a few who had served jail terms for violent crimes and were small and nasty. So the total concentration doesn't tell you necessarily the make-up of the family. We look first at the total concentration because that's how we screen the population. But if someone comes in with bad family history, or they're a diabetic, we start delving into HDL and LDL. And if they've got a really ugly family history then we start looking at LDL particle size and other things that can give us a clue as to where the real problem is. There's lots of further testing that can be performed.'

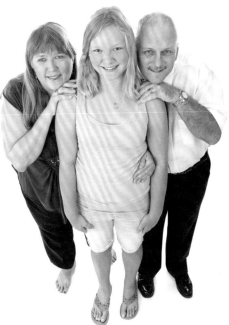

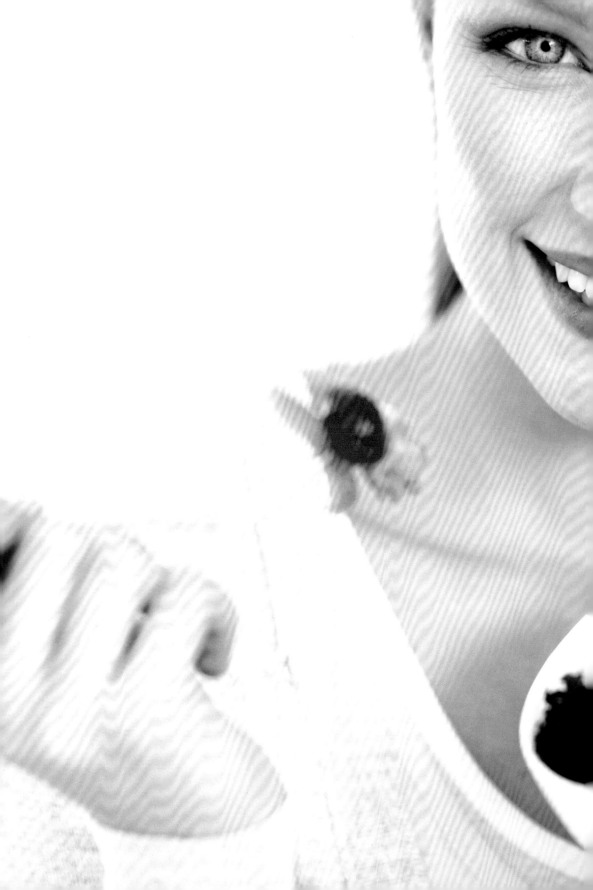

Treatments

When designing a treatment and management plan for a patient with high blood pressure and cholesterol, we've ascertained that it's essential to gather information beyond the condition the patient presents with and to look for other risks that they may also have. Professor Ian Meredith says that using context to help establish the patient's overall and absolute risks is the first step to building an effective treatment plan. So to recap, a 40-year-old woman who is a non-smoker, is not overweight, has no family history of heart disease and is fit and healthy except for slightly-elevated blood pressure would probably not be administered blood pressure-lowering medications off the bat. The doctor might prescribe a little more exercise per week and tweaks to her diet, and in all likelihood, they would be sufficient. The woman's overall and absolute risks were low. But if that woman's neighbour presented with a slightly raised blood pressure, yet she was a smoker, enjoyed a couple of glasses of wine each night and had lost her parent to a heart attack at age forty-five, then she would be offered a vastly different treatment plan - one that may well include medications.

When you're trying to get your high blood pressure and cholesterol under control, unless you've been assessed as needing pharmacological intervention, lifestyle changes work well. Diet, exercise and minimising exposure to tobacco smoke should be the major focus as they can help to lower your levels.

Diet

While diet can certainly help to reduce high cholesterol, it should be noted that major international studies consistently conclude that diet can only reduce your cholesterol levels by about 10 per cent and that genetic factors are far more powerful than a good diet.

'I think that instead of getting into these massive food wars where we debate what is good, what isn't good, what lowers your cholesterol, what's proven and what's not proven, the easiest way to do this is if you look at the really big studies of dietary intervention,' Professor Meredith explains. 'Those huge studies consistently find that dietary interventions only lower blood cholesterol by 10 per cent. That's about as big an effect that they can have. In any one individual you might get a 15 per cent or a

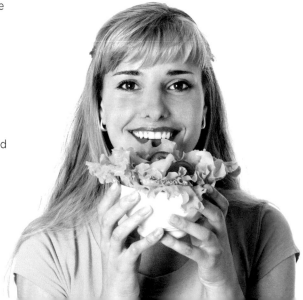

20 per cent cholesterol lowering, but if you took 10,000 people, their cholesterol would reduce on average by about 10 per cent and after a year, it'll be about seven per cent. So it's not a big impact. If you're a person of high absolute risk of heart disease, and you've got high cholesterol and need to reduce it by 50 per cent, you're not going to be able to do that just with diet modification. Having said that, diet should be the underpinning. You can't take a tablet and say, "OK I can eat cream buns". It' doesn't offset that. And, a 10 per cent difference can be quite significant for many people so by no means am I suggesting diet modification is not an effective cholesterol-lowering tool. What I am saying is that genetics are more powerful and your cholesterol level is mostly genetically-determined.

'People come to see me with high cholesterol and tell me, "I don't eat this and I don't eat that yet I have high cholesterol". Well that's just bad luck. Your cholesterol is high for other reasons. They come in to my rooms and they say they've got high cholesterol, but they don't eat this and they don't eat that, so why on earth would their reading be high? I tell them, "Yes, but you've got grey hair". There's often a look of confusion at that point. There's no association between cholesterol and hair colour, but that's exactly what I'm saying. If you came to my rooms and I said that your hair is grey, you wouldn't then say to me, "but I don't eat this and I don't eat that" because you don't believe there's any association between diet and the colour of your hair. Once you establish that the relationship between what you eat and your cholesterol level is somewhat tenuous, and that you're only modifying it a little bit, people get it.'

While you can't do much about your genetics, you can work on your diet, and you can achieve significant results. Reducing salt in your diet and eating a heart-healthy diet with lots of fresh fruit and vegetables is recommended, as is introducing foods containing omega 3 fatty acids and antioxidants. Animal-based products should be limited.

'Fish oil, on the whole, probably works so we would encourage people to have a high fish diet because the omega 3 fatty acids are good for you,' Professor Meredith says. 'Diets that are high in fresh fruit and vegetables seem to lower your blood pressure and so does reducing your salt intake.

'But the message I always share with people is to eat things that come from plants and animals, not things made in a plant. And you should eat more plants than animals. If you eat more plants than animals and things not made in a plant, you'll probably do very well in terms of your long-term health. And the less cooked the better.

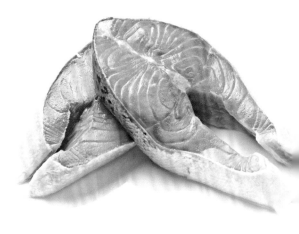

'All green vegetables are good for you. If it's brightly coloured and it's a fruit or veg then you should eat it because it contains natural antioxidants. Most of those bright colours come from molecules that have antioxidant-type potentials. And fish oil has positive effects on the platelets, the clotting elements of the blood, and it probably affects the triglycerides and the HDL a little bit. It may even lower the nervous drive to the body a little. There's evidence to support that and it very well might have modest blood pressure lowering effect.'

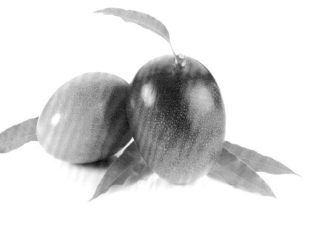

Nutritional Therapist and NutriLife Clinic founder Janine Fahri agrees that diet modification is an effective tool to help lower cholesterol and blood pressure.

'There are specific things you could eat to help lower your cholesterol and others you should avoid if you have high cholesterol,' she says.

'In terms of specific foods to avoid if your cholesterol is elevated and you're trying to lower it, the thing I say to my patients is to cut out foods that are high in saturated and hydrogenated fats. So I say a flat out no to things like biscuits, burgers, butter, cakes, too much cheese, chips, crisps, cream and creamy sauces, fatty, fried and oily foods, Greek yoghurt (because it's high in saturated fat), ice cream, lard, margarine, pastries, pepperoni and salami – things people don't really think about – as well as pies, pizza, poultry skin, processed food, sausages, streaky bacon, any white visible fat on red meat and whole milk. Those are the things I just say an outright 'no' to. They're not good for you anyway, before you even consider blood pressure and cholesterol.

'Then there are foods that I'd suggest you do your best to avoid – refined grains, for example. So that's your white bread, rice and pasta. Also, sweets and chocolate. And, if you haven't already eliminated them from your diet because they're high in saturated fats, cakes and biscuits. A low sugar diet has been shown to reduce blood cholesterol and plasma lipids, or fats, in the blood.
'I'd also recommend avoiding stimulants including tea, coffee and fizzy drinks because they have an impact on weight control, which in turn affects blood cholesterol.'

Interestingly, foods naturally high in cholesterol need not be avoided, Ms Fahri suggests.

'There are lots of people out there who think that they can't eat foods like eggs and seafood because they are foods naturally high in cholesterol,' she says. 'But there's no conclusive evidence out there that when you eat cholesterol it affects your blood cholesterol levels. It's the foods high in saturated fats that have that blood cholesterol level-raising effect but I still err on the side of caution and recommend not having too much of those food types anyway. I believe everything should be eaten in moderation. A healthy diet is a varied diet.

'As for foods you should increase in your diet to avoid high cholesterol, they are foods that contain essential fats.'

Foods containing essential fats include: avocado, brazil nuts, canola oil, flaxseeds, hemp seeds, oily fish like salmon, mackerel, anchovies, sardines, herring and fresh tuna (but not canned tuna as the canning process removes its beneficial qualities), pumpkin seeds, walnuts and dark leafy greens like kale and spinach.

Ms Fahri recommends two pieces of fruit and a minimum of three vegetables every day. 'Plus, I tell my patients who are trying to lower their cholesterol to have at least one apple or pear a day, because they contain soluble fibre, which assists in the elimination of cholesterol from the body.'

So, an apple a day may in fact keep the doctor away. Apple contains soluble fibre, which assists with the elimination of cholesterol from the body.

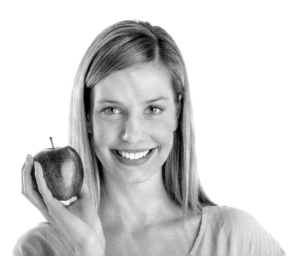

The fruits that may assist to lower cholesterol are:
apples, apricots, blackberries, blueberries, cherries, citrus fruits, melon, nectarines, pears, pineapple and strawberries.
'And go for organic whenever you can,' Ms Fahri suggests.

'It's the fibre content in these fruits and veg that make them particularly beneficial. One of the best things you can eat to help lower cholesterol is avocado. Half an avocado a day has been shown to lower your cholesterol by as much as two points in four months, primarily because of the beta-sitosterol it contains. Now obviously you can't have a poor diet and then eat half an avocado a day and expect it to lower your cholesterol by two points. A healthy eating plan should be used in conjunction with other lifestyle modifications to lower your cholesterol levels.'

Vegetables shown to be effective for lowering cholesterol include:
broccoli, brussel sprouts, carrots, cauliflower, kale, leeks, onions, capsicums, spinach, tomatoes and watercress.

'But the really good vegetables to help lower cholesterol are artichokes and beetroot,' Ms Fahri says. 'And beetroot can be really effective for helping to lower blood pressure too. In fact, studies show that drinking 500ml of nitrate-rich beetroot juice daily can improve heart function, lower blood pressure by as much as 10 per cent and increase exercise performance.'

Other foods that are a good source of fibre, and therefore effective when trying to lower cholesterol are: apples, brown rice and red rice, multigrain bread, sugarfree mueseli, peas, rye bread, sweetcorn, wholemeal bread and whole grains.

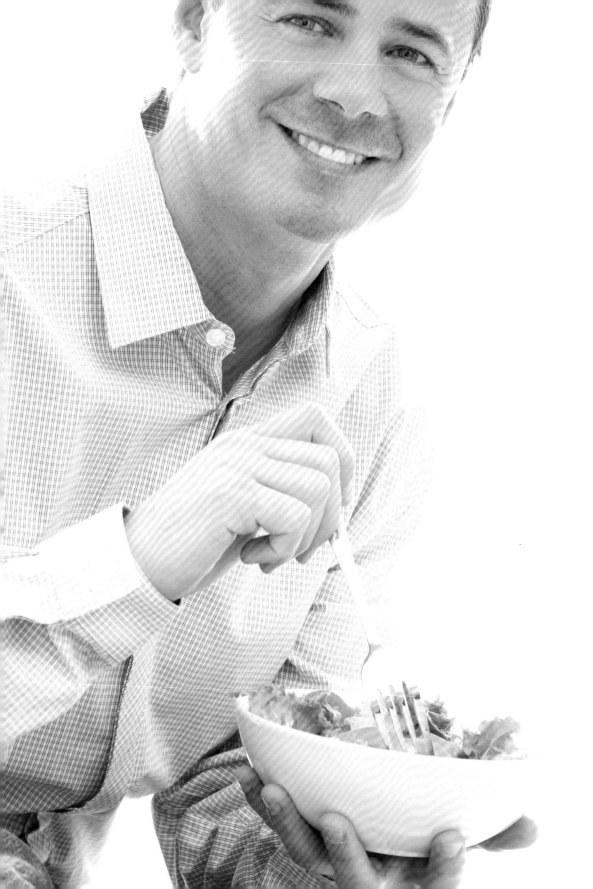

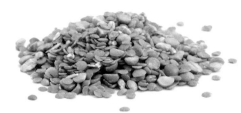

'And I also recommend bran and pulses like black-eyed peas, butter beans, peas, lentils and red kidney beans,' Ms Fahri says. 'And vitamin B3 has also been found in some studies to lower bad cholesterol by as much as 20-30 per cent and increase good cholesterol by about the same amount.'

Foods rich in B3 are:
halibut, mushrooms, natural peanuts, sunflower seeds and fresh and wild organic tuna.

However, it should be noted that other studies, including the Heart Protection Study - a mammoth controlled-randomised study undertaken to ascertain whether vitamins help to modify cardiovascular risk - found that vitamins made little or moderate difference to cardiovascular risk. More information about the Heart Protection Study will feature later in this chapter.

Ms Fahri recommends that diet modification should go hand-in-hand with other lifestyle changes in order to effectively lower blood pressure and cholesterol.

'Besides including some of these good foods in their diets and avoiding the bad ones, I would also recommend my patients engage in regular exercise. Not necessarily intense cardiovascular exercise like running, but perhaps brisk walking.'

With an academic background in psychology, Ms Fahri also confidently advocates employing stress management techniques to help with not only lowering blood pressure and cholesterol, but for general wellbeing.

'I strongly recommend the use of stress management techniques, as stress can be a factor directly and indirectly for high blood pressure and for raising cholesterol,' Ms Fahri says.

'And I'd also recommend my patients have an adrenal stress profile test. If you've got high stress levels or low thyroid function, both of those can raise cholesterol levels.

'For stress management, I advocate Pilates, yoga, tai chi, meditation and aromatherapy. I tell my patients to book in for reflexology, a facial or a massage and encourage everyone to have an hour a day of 'me-time'. These are all great stress relievers.'

A cholesterol and blood pressure-lowering action plan should also take alcohol consumption into consideration.

'Excessive alcohol can raise your blood pressure because it can contribute to weight gain. It also depletes nutrients and disrupts blood sugar regulation, and that can trigger cholesterol production,' Ms Fahri explains. 'It also adds to the burden on your liver, which then hinders the body's detoxification process and the clearance of cholesterol from the system. However, there are some studies that show a glass of wine a day can lower cholesterol because of its antioxidant properties. But it should be made clear that only one standard 150ml glass of red wine is acceptable. Even so, I wouldn't recommend a glass of wine or include it in a cholesterol-lowering program because you can get the same antioxidant benefits from eating things like blueberries instead.'

In summary, modifications to your diet can help to reduce high blood pressure, and cholesterol can be lowered by an average of 10 per cent by adopting a healthy diet, rich in cholesterol-lowering foods. The most effective dietary changes include:

- reducing salt
- including fish oil and foods rich in omega 3 fatty acids
- eating brightly-coloured fruits and vegetables that are high in antioxidants
- eating a varied diet containing both plant and animal-based foods
- avoiding foods high in saturated and hydrogenated fats
- avoiding refined grains
- avoiding stimulants like tea, coffee and fizzy drinks
- modifying consumption of cholesterol-rich foods
- eating foods that contain essential fats
- eating organic foods whenever possible
- eating foods high in fibre
- eating foods rich in Vitamin B3
- reducing alcohol consumption

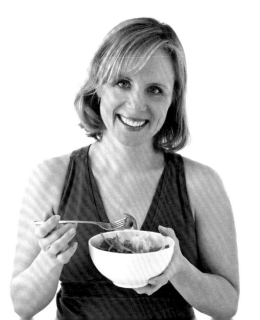

Exercise

According to the American Heart Foundation, adopting a healthy lifestyle is critical for the prevention of high blood pressure and high cholesterol, and an indispensable part of managing them. It recommends viewing these healthy lifestyle changes as a 'lifestyle prescription'.

While eating a better diet is one of the recommended major lifestyle changes, exercise and physical activity is another. Exercise not only assists with a healthy heart, it helps with weight management, size of girth, it can be a stress reliever and it can also enhance the effectiveness of blood pressure medications.

'Exercise lowers blood pressure and there's fantastic evidence dating back many, many years showing that regular exercise lowers your blood pressure as effectively as a single blood pressure medication,' Professor Ian Meredith advises. 'If you're taking a single line hypertensive agent, just one, you can pretty much achieve the same effect with thirty to forty minutes of brisk walking three or four times a week. It's a no-brainer. Obviously weight reduction, reducing alcohol, reducing salt and things like yoga, Pilates and tai chi probably do contribute to a reasonable burden of blood pressure that people can actually modify. When it comes to cholesterol, unfortunately that is mainly genetically determined, and a high natural blood cholesterol level, well that's just bad luck. But exercise can definitely help.'

About 150 minutes of moderate-intensity aerobic physical activity per week, and engaging in muscle strengthening activities more than two days a week can help to lower cholesterol.

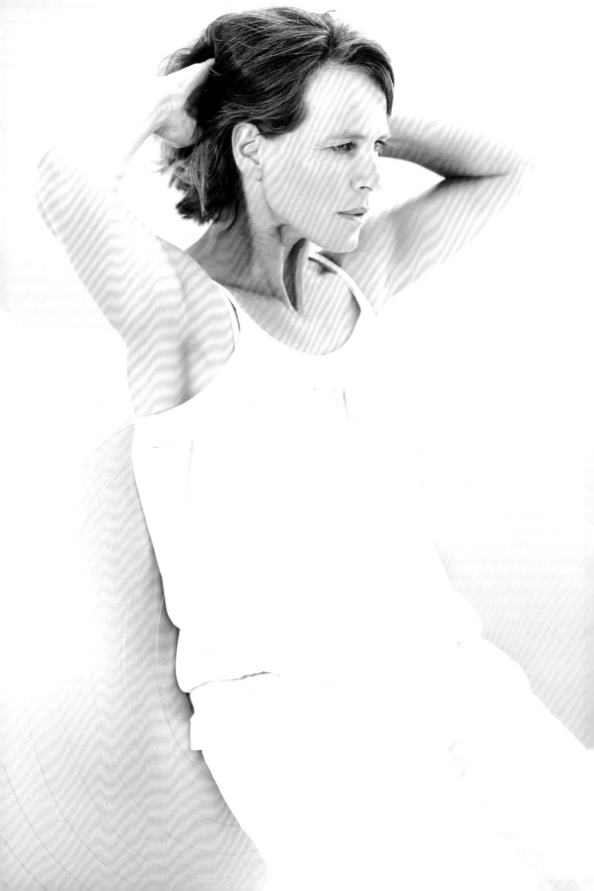

Pharmacological

Statins are among the biggest-selling medications worldwide. They are a class of drug used to lower cholesterol levels by inhibiting the enzyme HMG-CoA reductase, which plays an instrumental role in the production of cholesterol in the liver. Our liver produces about 70 per cent of the body's total cholesterol. As we've learned, high cholesterol levels can lead to cardiovascular disease.

'You can't not have a discussion on cholesterol without talking about statins, fibrates, ezetrol and things like that,' Professor Meredith says. 'You need to put statins into context. They are medications and, yes, they do have side effects but the body of evidence to support them is pretty fantastic. Statins are to cardiovascular disease in the second half of the 21st century what antibiotics were to infection in the first half of the 20th century. They're amazing things, but like all things, they come with down sides and risks. They have to be used appropriately, but they have undoubtedly a major impact on reducing the risks particularly in people with established heart disease. They're a very important treatment but taking these medications is not a set-and-forget strategy.'

The Heart Protection Study

The Heart Protection Study involved 20,000 subjects in the UK and was a trial that studied the use of statin medication and vitamin supplementation (vitamin E, vitamin C and beta carotene) in patients who were at risk of cardiovascular disease.

'It was a, double-blind, placebo-controlled randomised trial by the British Heart Foundation and the Medical Research Council, and its data was analysed by Rory Collins and colleagues at Oxford University. So it was completely independent and beautifully done,' Professor Meredith says. 'There was a five-year follow-up, 10,000 in each arm, against placebo and it found that there's a minimum 30 per cent difference in the outcome of the people who are on statin treatment versus those not on treatment. There are a million other cholesterol studies that conclude the same.'

'In cholesterol management, diet is the number one strategy, getting rid of all the other risk factors,' Professor Meredith says. 'Then, beyond that, once lifestyle changes have been implemented, or if there's cause to go down the medication route immediately, statins are the key thing where appropriate. For some patients, you can use other medications like fibrates, or medications such as cholestyramine, or bile salt sequestrants.

Bile salts are made of cholesterol, which are excreted in your faeces. So with bile salt sequestrants, your bile salt is eliminated and you therefore have to make more bile, which means you use up more of your body's cholesterol in order to do that. It's an old-fashioned treatment, but it does work. Other treatments are ezetrol or ezetimibe, which are cholesterol absorption inhibitors, niacin and cholestyramine, a bile acid sequestrant.'

Cholesterol medications

Statins (HMG CoA reductase inhibitors)

This class of drugs works in the liver to prevent the formation of cholesterol. Statins are most effective at lowering the LDL (bad) cholesterol, but they also have a minor positive effect on lowering triglycerides (blood fats) and raising HDL (good) cholesterol.

Selective cholesterol absorption inhibitors

This class of cholesterol-lowering medications has been around since the early 2000s and works by preventing the absorption of cholesterol from the intestine. Selective cholesterol absorption inhibitors, like statins, are most effective at lowering the LDL cholesterol, but they only have a modest effect on lowering triglycerides and raising HDL cholesterol.

Resins - also known as bile acid sequestrants or bile acid-binding drugs

Resins work in the intestines by helping to increase the disposal of cholesterol. The body uses cholesterol to make bile, an acid used during digestion. This cholesterol-lowering class of drug binds to bile so it can't be used during digestion. So your body makes more bile in response. The more bile your liver makes, the more cholesterol is used up, so there is less cholesterol left to circulate through blood.

Lipid-lowering Therapies

Fibrates (fibric acid derivatives): These are best at lowering triglycerides and can sometimes have a positive impact on HDL levels. These drugs are not very effective in lowering LDL cholesterol, which is why they are generally used in people whose triglycerides are high or whose HDL is low, after reaching LDL goal. Fibrates can be used in combination therapy with statins.

Niacin (nicotinic acid): This drug works in the liver by affecting the production of blood fats. Niacin is prescribed to lower triglycerides and LDL cholesterol and raise HDL cholesterol.

Niacin comes in prescription form and as dietary supplements. The dietary supplement version of niacin must not be used as a substitute for prescription niacin as there are potential serious side effects.

Omega-3 Fatty Acid Ethyl Esters are derived from fish oils that are chemically changed and purified and are used in combination with diet modification to lower high levels of triglycerides.

Marine-Derived Omega-3 Polyunsaturated Fatty Acids (PUFA), known as omega-3 fish oils or omega-3 fatty acids, are used in large doses to lower high triglyceride levels in the blood. They help decrease triglyceride secretion and facilitate triglyceride clearance. It's difficult to attain enough of these to make a difference from diet alone so supplementation may be prescribed by your doctor.

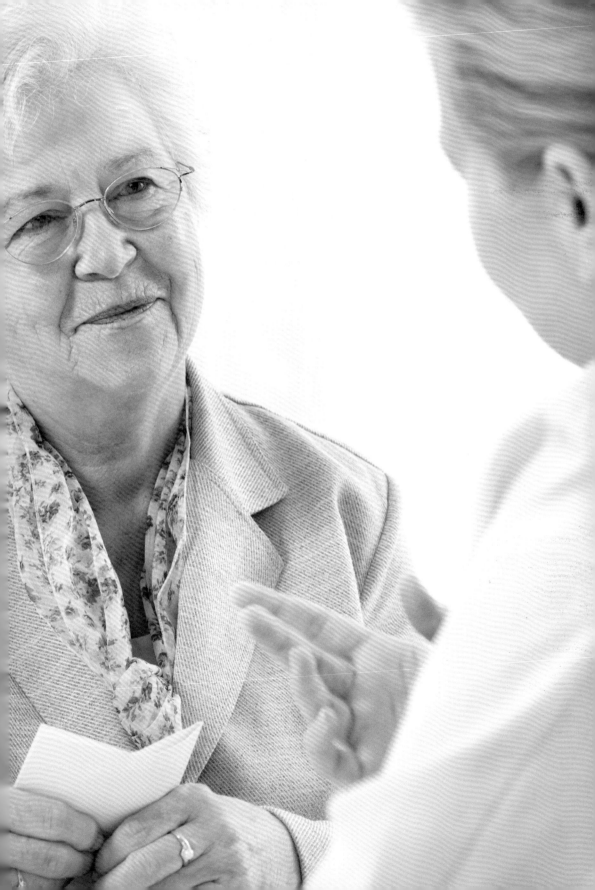

Known side effects of cholesterol medications

Most side effects of statins are mild and generally go away as your body adjusts but there are rare reports of muscle problems and liver abnormalities. As a precaution, your doctor may order regular liver function tests. Patients who are pregnant or who have active or chronic liver disease should not take statins.

Possible side effects:

Muscle pain and muscle damage is the most common statin-use side effect and may involve soreness, tiredness or weakness in your muscles. The pain might be mild or severe enough to affect your daily activities. On rare occasions, statins can cause life-threatening muscle damage called rhabdomyolysis (rab-doe-mi-OL-ih-sis), which can cause severe muscle pain, liver damage, kidney failure and death. Rhabdomyolysis can occur when you take statins in combination with certain drugs or if you take a high dose of statins.

Liver damage may occur with statin use. Occasionally, statins can cause your liver to increase its production of enzymes that help you digest food, drinks and medications. Although liver problems are rare, your doctor will likely order a liver enzyme test before or shortly after you start taking a statin. Signs of an issue include unusual fatigue or weakness, loss of appetite, pain in your upper abdomen, dark-colored urine, or yellowing of your skin or eyes.

Digestive problems may also be an issue. Nausea, gas, diarrhea or constipation may occur after taking a statin. These side effects are rare for people with normal digestive systems. Taking statin medication after your evening meal can reduce digestive side effects.

You might develop a rash or flushing after you start taking a statin. Aspirin might help but seeking a doctor's advice is necessary before taking any additional medications.

There's a small chance that your blood sugar (blood glucose) level may increase when you take a statin, which may lead to developing type 2 diabetes.

Neurological side effects have also been reported from statin use, including memory loss and confusion. These side effects reverse once you stop taking the medication. There has also been evidence that statins may help with brain function in patients with dementia or Alzheimer's and studies are underway. It is crucial not to stop taking your statin medication before seeking your doctor's advice.

Known side effects of cholesterol medications

Niacin side effects

Niacin may cause flushing, itching and stomach upset. Your liver functions may be closely monitored, as niacin can cause toxicity. Non-prescription immediate-release forms of niacin usually have the most side effects, especially at higher doses. Niacin is also used cautiously in diabetic patients as it can raise blood sugar levels.

Marine-derived omega-3 PUFA side effects

In large doses, these may cause serious side effects including increased bleeding, hemorrhagic stroke and reduced blood sugar control in diabetics and they may interact negatively with other medications, herbal preparations and nutritional supplements. Individuals with allergies to fish and/or shellfish may have a severe adverse reaction to use of these supplements.

Source: Mayo Clinic

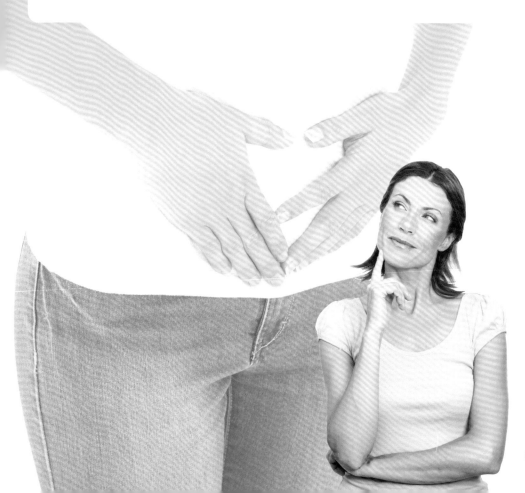

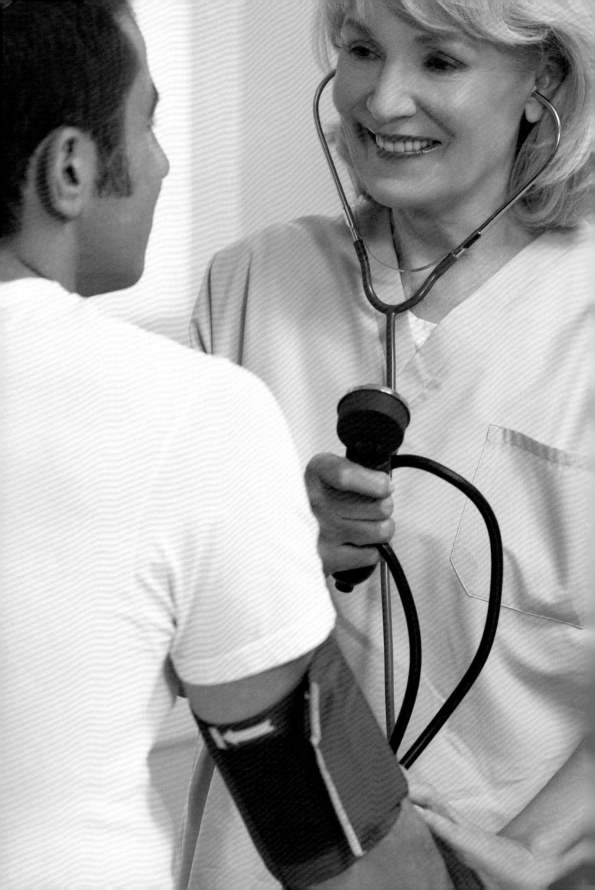

Treatment of blood pressure, like cholesterol treatment, also begins with non-pharmacological methods.

'In order of treating blood pressure, firstly you always start with non-pharmacological treatments – diet, exercise, stopping smoking and all the things we've covered. Second, you rule out all preventative and reversible causes of high blood pressure, because sometimes people have reversible causes of hypertension, like coarctation of the aorta, narrowing to a kidney artery, high calcium levels, and excess adrenal production of the hormones, each of which might be correctible. They're what we call secondary causes of hypertension, so we need to blow those out. And then, after all those options are exhausted, there's a range of blood pressure medications, ACE inhibitors, diuretics, beta blockers, calcium antagonists, and vasodilators. They're the main classes and there are various forms of angiotensin receptor blockers. Which ones of these used, and in what combinations, depends entirely on the individual. But pharmacological therapy is only undertaken in the setting of consistently elevated, properly measured blood pressure and in the absence of secondary and preventable or reversible cause in conjunction with non-pharmacological therapy. Only then do you start pharmacological therapy and you choose which medications are best for each person; so an asthmatic wouldn't use a beta blocker, or if you've got a kidney problem you might not use a diuretic.'

When exploring pharmacological intervention for lowering blood pressure and cholesterol, aspirin should also be considered, according to Professor Meredith.

'Aspirin also fits in the picture for people who have established risk profile or established heart disease and there's a study called the Aspirin Triallists Collaboration where all the studies ever undertaken on aspirin, in massive analyses of hundreds of thousands of people, are assessed. The ten-year benefit of being on aspirin if you have established heart disease is that it reduces your risk of recurrent events by about 20 per cent. But, should a forty-year-old who has high blood pressure on its own take aspirin? No, because it's not even clear that if the blood pressure is only moderately elevated that they should be on medications. You might send them out to do more exercise and eat more plants, and then check your blood pressure on a regular basis. Certainly pharmacological options should not be implemented without thorough analysis by your doctor.'

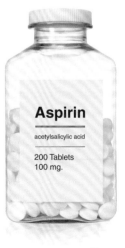

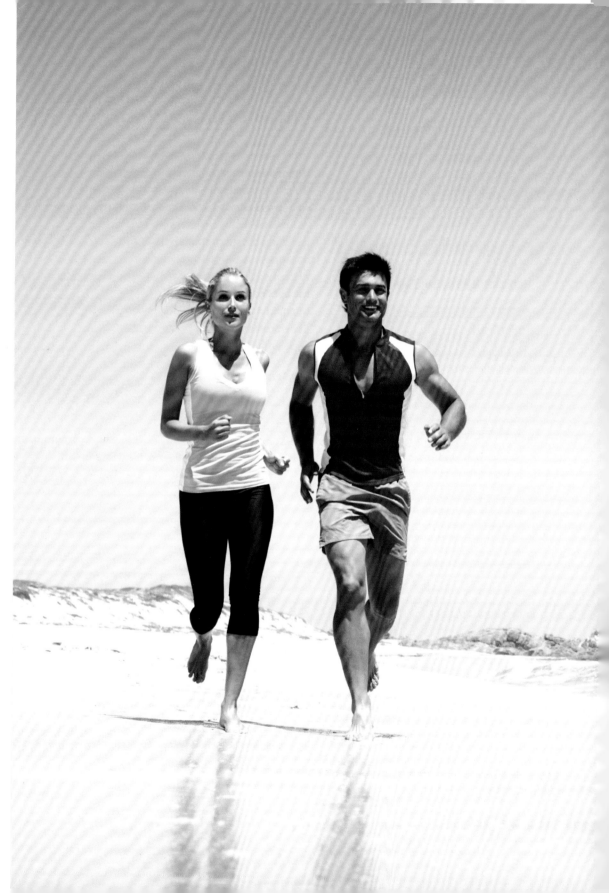

Tips for a healthy cholesterol level

1. Exercise for 30 minutes, five times a week.

No surprises here. Many research studies suggest that not only does moderate exercise decrease bad LDL cholesterol by five to ten per cent, it can also raise the body's good HDL cholesterol levels. Moderate exercise can include brisk walking but the more intense the aerobic exercises, like jogging, the more you can expect your HDL levels to rise. Current research indicates that 30 minutes of aerobic exercise can raise HDL levels by 3-6mg/dL. This rise is evident just 24 hours after exercising and can persist for up to fifteen days.

As most research into the effects of exercise on cholesterol have also investigated other cholesterol-lowering factors simultaneously, the true impact that exercise alone has on cholesterol hasn't been determined. However, recent studies that have focused specifically on the relationship between cholesterol and exercise have been revealing. Studies have shown that exercise can affect the size of your lipoproteins. LDL, as we know, are associated with causing cardiovascular disease (CVD). Moderate exercise can increase the size of your LDL particles, which reduces that CVD risk. Early studies also suggest that exercise can improve the transportation of cholesterol from the rest of the body to the liver, where cholesterol is expelled from the body. Furthermore, researchers have found that eight to twelve weeks of endurance exercise may slightly reduce the absorption of cholesterol from the small intestine into the blood. Exercise does not appear to influence the actual amount of cholesterol that the liver produces, however.

2. Exercise for fifteen-minute intervals

If you're time poor and can't manage regular thirty-minute workouts, some studies have concluded that the same healthy benefits are possible by dividing this exercise time into fifteen-minute intervals.

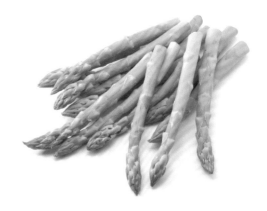

3. Lose weight

Again, this isn't rocket science. Obesity goes hand-in-hand with low HDL and high LDL. Foods like fish, vegetable oils and whole grains can raise HDLs and lower LDL, and these are food types usually found in weight loss diet plans. LDL is raised when you consume foods containing saturated fats like butter, whole fat dairy and red meat. These are the type of foods usually forbidden from healthy eating plans, so losing weight certainly helps improve HDL levels and reduces LDL.

4. Increase your vitamin B intake

Niacin is a B vitamin that's used by the body to turn carbohydrates into energy, and it's also been found to increase HDL and moderately decrease LDL and triglycerides. While most people eat enough niacin through their diet to effectively turn carbs into energy, unfortunately, you can't consume enough niacin through food to get the HDL-raising effect. Niacin is available in supplement form, and on prescription for those with niacin deficiency or to increase HDL cholesterol. You must not take an over-the-counter niacin supplement without first talking to your doctor as there can be serious side effects.

5. Eat cold-water fish at least twice a week

The American Heart Association recommends eating at least two servings of fatty fish a week, like salmon, mackerel, lake trout, herring, sardines and halibut, because they contain high levels of omega-3 fatty acid called docosahexaenoic acid (DHA). DHA helps to raise good HDL cholesterol, while also protecting brain health, eye health and helping to reduce blood pressure.

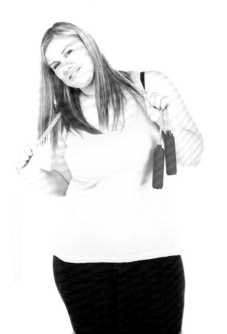

6. Introduce an algae-based omega-3 supplement

To ensure you get plenty of DHA to impact HDL levels, an algae-based omega-3 supplement may also be taken after consultation with your doctor. But it's worth noting that you shouldn't simply substitute a supplement for fresh fish as there are additional nutritional benefits from eating fresh fish, like selenium, that are not present in omega-3 supplements.

7. Bake or grill fish

If you do add fish to your diet, make sure you don't negate the positives by cooking it in an unhealthy way. Bake or grill fish as opposed to frying it to avoid adding unhealthy fats.

8. Use ground flaxseed or canola oil for an omega-3 boost

IIf you don't like fish, you can get a small amount of omega-3 fatty acids from ground flaxseed or canola oil. Flaxseed can help to lower your cholesterol and it's better to use ground flaxseed as the body digests it better.

9. Flaxseed tips

To add flaxseed to your diet, mix a tablespoon of ground flaxseed into yoghurt or your breakfast cereal. You can even add a teaspoon to mayonnaise or mustard. You'll barely notice.

10. Go nuts!

Rich in polyunsaturated fatty acids, nuts - including walnuts, almonds, pistachios, hazelnuts, pecans, peanuts and some pine nuts - can help reduce blood cholesterol. You can eat a handful (about 40grams) a day to help with heart health, just make sure the nuts aren't salted or sugar-coated, and as they are high in calories, be careful that it is just a handful consumed.

11. Substitute nuts for foods high in saturated fats

Rich in polyunsaturated fatty acids, nuts To avoid weight gain, instead of eating foods high in saturated fats, substitute them with nuts. Try adding a handful of walnuts or almonds to a salad instead of cheese, meat or croutons.

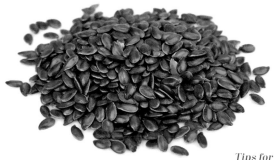

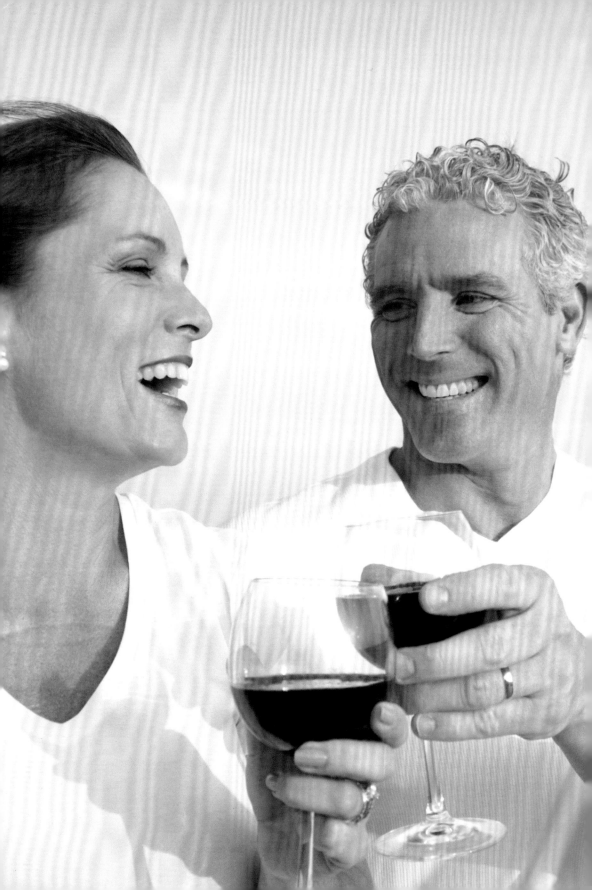

12. Stop smoking

The best thing you can do for heart health if you're a smoker is to give up the habit. It's no secret how damaging smoking can be and there are many, many research studies out there that conclude this. There is a chemical in cigarette called acrolein, which actually stops your HDL from transporting fatty deposits to the liver, which can ultimately lead to atherosclerosis, plaque build-up in the arteries and is the single biggest issue around high blood pressure and cholesterol. And a recent study by the Health Research Institute in Australia investigated why smoking affects good cholesterol. It was thought that the presence of certain oxidants in the bloodstream, which are elevated in smokers, may stop HDL from doing its job, resulting in the development of atherosclerosis.

13. Restrict alcohol intake

Ethanol in all forms of alcohol helps increase HDL cholesterol so a daily glass of red wine or other alcoholic drink may help to lower your risk of cardiovascular disease. But only one standard measure per day for women and two for men is considered an acceptable level. Grapes are a good source of antioxidant, so red wine is generally considered the better option. Red wine in particular is also beneficial for reducing the circulating levels of cholesterol in the blood. It also reduces the 'stickiness' of blood, especially at mealtimes, and improves the balance of good and bad cholesterols. But remember, it's a very fine line between the acceptable amount and too much.

14. Eat less sugar

Eating more than 90 grams of sugar each day can increase your bad LDL cholesterol and triglycerides while also reducing HDL. You should try to keep your added sugars to less than 100 calories per day, which equates to about two tablespoons. You might be surprised where you can find hidden added sugar. Cereals are notoriously high, as are condiments like tomato sauce, sweet chilli sauce and barbecue sauce, and salad dressings are surprisingly high too. Processed foods contain a heap of sugar so take it easy and certainly avoid adding your own sprinkling of sugar on top.

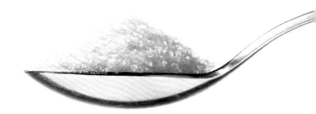

15. Reduce foods high in saturated fat

Unhealthy saturated fat and trans fat raise LDL, and trans fats reduce HDL too. By cutting down on your meat intake and full-fat dairy, you can lessen the impact. No more than seven per cent of your daily calories should come from saturated fat. Don't include processed foods – like chips, sweet and savoury biscuits and margarine - in your diet, or anything containing partially hydrogenated vegetable oils. Substitute chips for a handful of nuts, and have skim milk on your cereal rather than full-cream milk.

16. Avoid palm and coconut oils

Unhealthy saturated fat and trans fat raise While most vegetable oils are unsaturated, there are a couple that contain mostly saturated fat – palm oil and coconut oil. Instead of these two, choose unsaturated varieties like sunflower, canola, safflower, corn, olive, soybean and peanut oils.

17. Read food labels

A great tip for reducing unwanted nasties in your diet is to read food labels carefully. Food contents are listed in order of prevalence so if prepared food packaging lists products like meat fat, coconut or palm oil, cream, butter, egg or yolk solids, whole milk solids, lard, cocoa butter, chocolate or imitation chocolate, or hydrogenated or partially hydrogenated fat or oil early in the listing, try to avoid it as they are the predominant ingredients.

18. Avoid fast foods that have no food labels

Foods that are not labelled should probably be consumed sparingly because it's difficult to make an assessment as to whether they are good or bad for you.

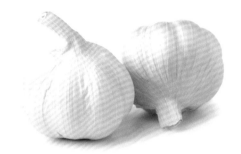

19. Eat more garlic

Studies reveal that eating garlic as part of a low-fat diet can help to reduce bad LDL levels and raise good HDL cholesterol. Garlic also helps to thin the blood, which reduces risk of heart attack. In countries where more garlic is consumed, there is a lower rate of heart disease.

20. Increase your legume intake

Legumes, including lentils, chickpeas, beans and peas, have a positive effect on bad LDL. You can add them to soups or salads, and you wouldn't even realise they were there if you put them in stews and casseroles, even if you're not a fan of the flavours. They are low in fat and rich in nutrients like B vitamins and they are a great source of soluble fibre, which helps to lower cholesterol levels. A study from Arizona State University found that subjects who consumed half a cup of beans a day over 24 weeks lowered their cholesterol by eight per cent.

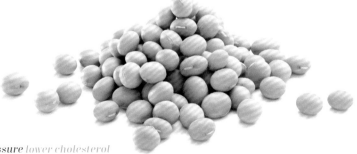

21. Reduce the amount of animal fat in your diet

Possibly the most effective way to reduce your cholesterol is to reduce the amount of animal fat in your diet. Found in anything that comes from an animal – meats, poultry, egg yolks, cheese and whole milks – animal fats are complex mixtures of triglycerides with lesser amounts of phospholipids and cholesterol. So all foods containing animal fat contain cholesterol.

22. Eat porridge/ oatmeal for breakfast

Adding foods that have high quantities of soluble fibre to your diet can help to lower your LDL. Soluble fibre can reduce the absorption of cholesterol into your bloodstream so eating porridge or oatmeal for breakfast can decrease your bad cholesterol level. You need to consume five to ten grams or more of soluble fibre per day for it to have a cholesterol-lowering effect. One-and-a-half cups of oatmeal provides about six grams, so if you add fibre-rich fruit to your morning meal, like pear, apple, banana or prunes, you'll well and truly meet the recommended level.

23. Eat two tablespoons of olive oil a day

Olive oil contains antioxidants that can help to lower LDL cholesterol without affecting your good HDL cholesterol. In place of other fats in your diet, use two tablespoons of olive oil to gain its heart-healthy benefits. Try gently cooking vegetables in olive oil, mixing it with vinegar as a salad dressing or making a marinade out of it. Rather than spreading butter on bread, dip bread in olive oil. Like nuts, olive oil is high in calories so don't use more than two tablespoons a day.

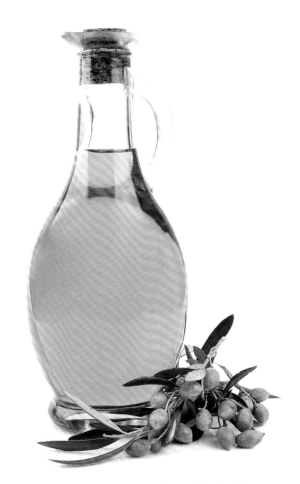

24. Choose extra virgin olive oil over regular olive oil

Extra virgin olive oil has not been processed as much as regular olive oil so has more antioxidants and its cholesterol-lowering effects are therefore greater. Be aware though that olive oils labelled 'light' are processed even more than regular olive oils. Light refers to its colour, not that it's lower in fat or calories.

25. Eat food with added plant sterols or stanols

Sterols or stanols are substances found in plants that help to block the absorption of cholesterol into your bloodstream. There are now foods on the market that have been fortified with sterols and stanols, including margarines, orange juice and yoghurt drinks. You need at least two grams of plant sterols in your diet each day to help reduce your LDL cholesterol by as much as ten per cent.

26. Eat half an avocado per day

Half an avocado a day in the context of a healthy eating plan has been shown to lower your cholesterol, primarily because of the beta-sitosterol it contains. Beta-sitosterol is a primary plant sterol.

27. Drink pomegranate juice

While there's no conclusive evidence that proves drinking pomegranate juice can lower your cholesterol, it is believed that pomegranate juice could block or slow the build-up of cholesterol in your arteries when you have elevated levels of fats in your blood and other heart disease risk factors. Pomegranate juice is rich in antioxidants, most notably polyphenols, which are thought to have heart-protecting properties, including lowering LDL. Make sure if you do choose to drink pomegranate juice that you're drinking pure juice and not a mixture of juices that contain added sugar.

28. Eat brightly-coloured vegetables

Bright vegetables contain natural antioxidants. Most of the bright colours come from molecules that have antioxidant-type potentials, so veg like carrots, broccoli, tomatoes, capsicums and Brussels sprouts. Antioxidants have heart-protecting benefits.

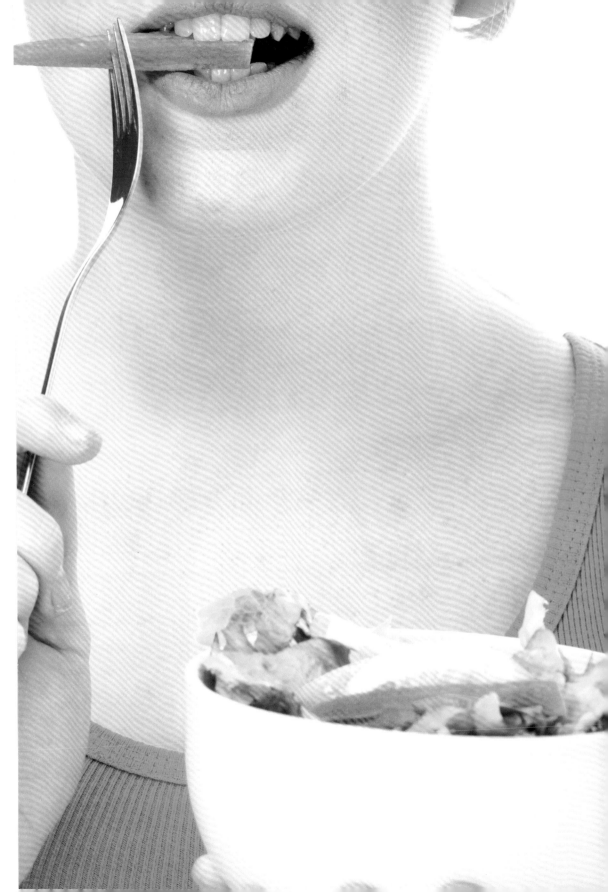

33. Snack on pistachios

When you get the 3pm munchies, make sure you have a handful of pistachios, or other cholesterol-lowering nuts like almonds and walnuts, handy so you aren't tempted to head over to the snack vending machine or grab a naughty snack from the coffee shop next door.

34. Park in the farthest corner of the car park

If you drive to work, park in the farthest corner of your car park to increase your incidental exercise. And try to take the stairs rather than the lift.

35. Hop off the train the station before your regular stop

If you catch public transport to work, disembark one stop earlier than usual and walk the rest of the way. Not only are you getting the cholesterol-lowering benefits of increased exercise, it'll get the blood flowing to the brain and you may find you're more productive once you arrive at work.

36. Split entrees in half

When dining out, if you order an entree, share it with your dining partner, or eat half and take the rest home. Restaurant portions are frequently two to three times larger than normal portions. Or, instead of ordering a main meal, order a salad or soup, which are often (but not always) a healthier option.

37. Serve dinner on smaller side plates instead of dinner plates

When eating at home, serve your meals on small side plates instead of large dinner plates. You can't pile as much food onto a smaller plate and it also tricks the brain into thinking it has a larger amount of food than it actually has.

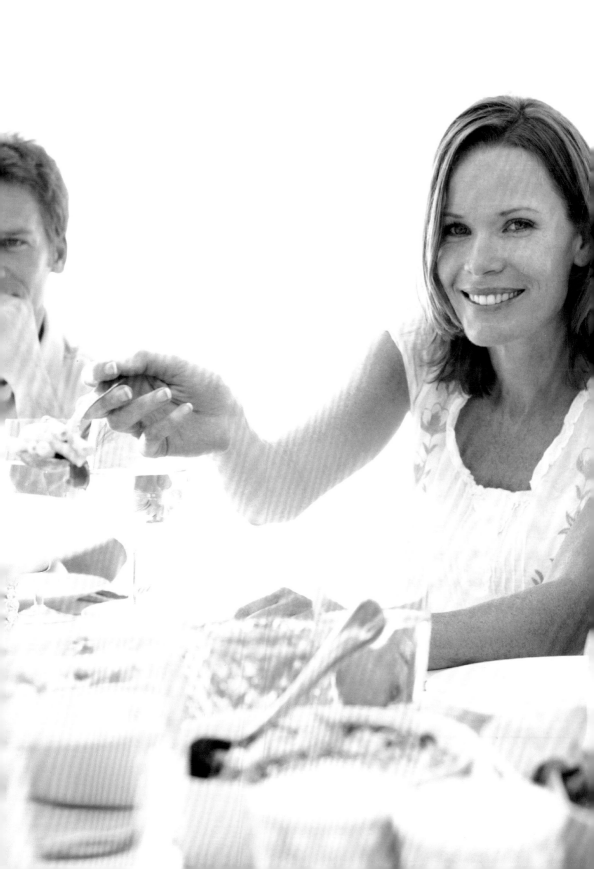

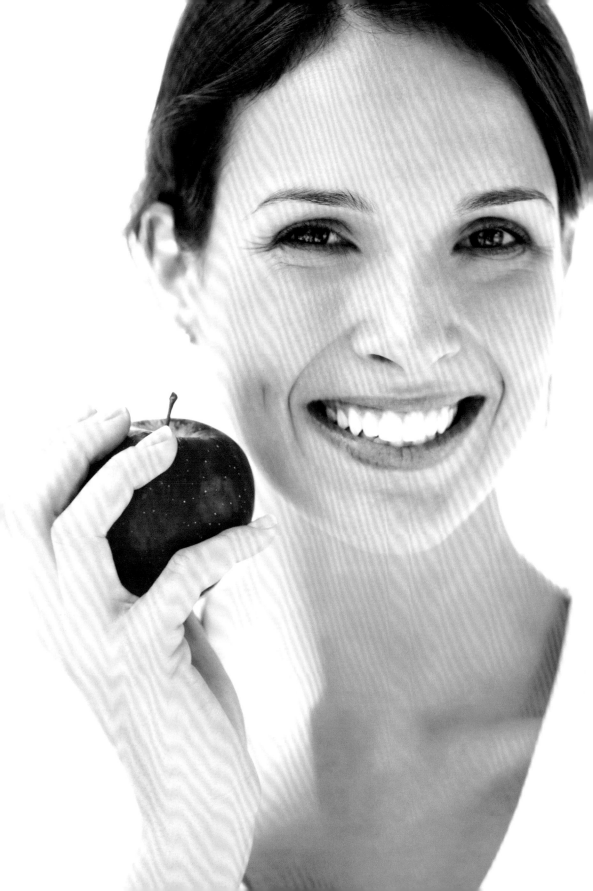

38. Avoid eating out of a carton or bag

Always remove food from its carton or bag, if that's how you buy it, and dish onto a small plate. It never ceases to amaze me how much food can be crammed into those small takeaway cartons. Eating from the container, you really can't tell just how much you're consuming. And as your brain only registers that you're full twenty minutes after you actually are, you probably eat way more than you need to if you eat straight out of the box.

39. Understand portion sizes

Reducing your portion sizes can have a heavy influence on your calorie consumption. These visuals can help you to know a little more about how big portions should be.

- Half a cup of vegetables is about the size of your fist
- A medium apple is the size of a cricket ball or baseball
- A serve of meat, fish or poultry is about 85 grams or the size of a deck of cards
- A serve of cheese is about 40 grams or the size of a pair of dice
- One tablespoon of butter is about the size of the tip of your thumb.

40. Eat an apple a day

A study published in the British Medical Journal compared the benefits of taking a statin a day with the benefits of eating an apple a day, like the old proverb suggests. Researchers from the British Heart Foundation Health Promotion Research Group at Oxford tested the health impact of both on study subjects aged 50-plus. They concluded that statins could prevent about 9500 British deaths from cardiovascular disease in the over 50s, while the folk remedy could prevent or delay about 8500 deaths. While the statins research group fared better, the impact of apples is undeniable. They are high in soluble fibre which assists in the elimination of cholesterol from the body. You shouldn't stop taking statins if your doctor has prescribed them. In fact, this study confirms that statins save lives.

41. Add beetroot to salads

Beetroots are full of carotenoids and flavenoids and studies have shown that they help lower and possibly even prevent the formation of LDL cholesterol in the body. Add beetroot to your salads or your sandwich. The health benefits outweigh the time it takes to remove the beetroot juice stains from your clothes.

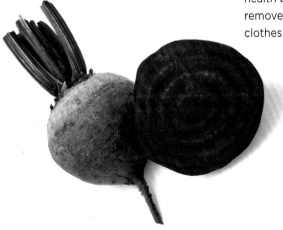

42. Add artichoke to your diet

Artichokes, which stimulate the flow of bile from the liver, have also been found in studies to have cholesterol-lowering properties. Add artichokes to your diet to enjoy their health benefits.

43. Talk to your family

Find out about your parents' health and that of your grandparents. If you have high cholesterol, you may not know about it as there are no side effects. Knowing if you're at a higher genetic risk of high cholesterol should prompt you to have a cholesterol test and make changes to reduce your levels if necessary.

44. Have healthy snacks

Keep little batons of chopped up carrot, cucumber, celery and capsicum in an airtight container and take them to work or pop them in your bag so when you get the mid-afternoon munchies you can snack on those rather than choosing an easy-grab, unhealthy option.

45. Know your fats

Educate yourself. Knowing which fats raise LDL cholesterol and which ones don't so you can modify your diet is one of the easiest ways to make changes to your cholesterol levels.

46. Avoid environments where people smoke

Studies have concluded that second-hand smoke can have the same effect on cholesterol levels as smoking itself. Avoid places where you'll be exposed to cigarette smoke to minimise your risk.

47. Join a walking group

Exercise undoubtedly helps to lower cholesterol levels. Joining a walking group can help to keep you motivated to exercise and being committed to a group means you're less likely to give the exercise a miss.

48. Make a pledge with loved ones

It's always easier making lifestyle changes if you're supported. Get your family and friends on board when trying to lower your cholesterol. Not only will it be easier cooking cholesterol-lowering foods that everyone in your family can eat, but family and friends can encourage the behavioural changes and perhaps won't bake those cupcakes next time you pop over for a visit.

49. Swap white bread for wholemeal or multigrain bread

Even making a simple dietary change like swapping white bread for multigrain or wholemeal bread can have a positive influence on your LDL. The grains in white bread have been refined, making it a less healthy alternative than multigrain or wholemeal breads, which contain good amounts of soluble fibre and therefore help with cholesterol reduction.

50. Have a massage/relaxation therapy

High stress levels have been linked to raised cholesterol. Have a massage, a facial, a foot rub, take a meditation or yoga class or even just take an hour away from the stresses of the day and sit on a beach or under a tree. Not only can it help to reduce stress and therefore cholesterol levels, it's a pat on the back for making positive changes to your health.

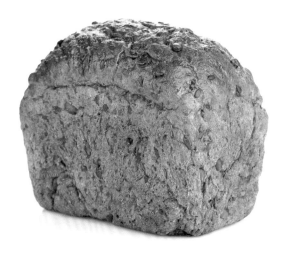

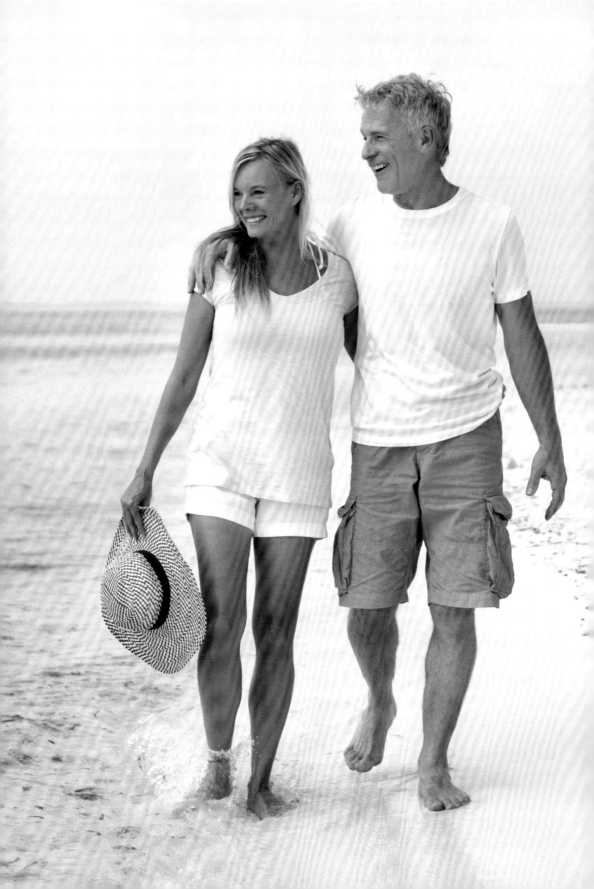

Tips for lowering your blood pressure

1. Take a brisk 30-minute walk each morning

Increasing your exercise to lower blood pressure is a no-brainer. The starting point of any blood pressure-lowering regime is encouraging a healthy lifestyle - increasing aerobic exercise, weight reduction (for every kilogram lost there's an average reduction of 1mmHg in blood pressure), reducing salt and restricting alcohol. If you have pre-hypertension, exercise can help you to avoid developing full-blown hypertension.

2. Keep a food diary

If you've never kept tabs on everything you eat before, you might be surprised to realise how much you do actually consume. Even keeping a food diary for a week can shed light on your dietary habits. The diary makes figuring out where your diet needs a tweak far easier.

3. Find one hidden source of salt a day and banish it from your diet

If you looked at the packaging on many foods, you might find salt as an ingredient where you didn't expect it. Breakfast cereal is a big one. Many common cereals contain salt. Swap to one that doesn't, or better still, a sugar-free muesli. Eliminating salt from your diet is one of the keys to dropping your blood pressure rate.

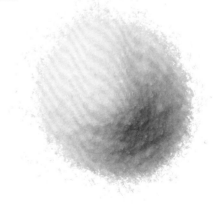

4. Don't add extra salt to your food

In one teaspoon of salt, there are 2300milligrams of sodium, which is the upper limit of what your daily intake of sodium should be for people below 50. Anyone with high blood pressure, diabetes, or chronic kidney disease - as well as African-Americans – should try to limit daily sodium intake to below 1500milligrams. Instead of adding salt, add other herbs and spices to boost the flavour of your food.

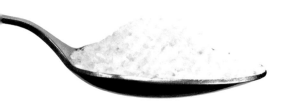

5. Have your blood pressure checked regularly

There are about 16 million people in the UK with high blood pressure but only around two-thirds of them know about it. Knowing you have a problem with blood pressure is half the battle. It often goes unnoticed because it's basically asymptomatic. When you visit the doctor, ask for your blood pressure to be checked. There are also some good automated blood pressure test kits available for home use but make sure it's reliable and validated so you're not misled. Having it checked professionally over a few visits to the doctor is the best way to ensure accuracy.

6. Boost your potassium intake

Fruits and vegetables are a great source of potassium. The best way to include more potassium into your diet is through food, rather than supplements, so making sure you eat at least five serves of fruit and veg a day should increase your potassium levels. Potassium has been shown to lessen the effects of sodium on blood. Your doctor can tell you what potassium level is best for you.

7. Add flaxseed to your food

Flaxseed is a fantastic plant source of omega-3 fatty acids, fibre and lignans – an antioxidant. However researchers of a recent study, published in the journal *Hypertension*, into the blood pressure-reducing benefits of linseeds are suggesting we add linseeds to our daily diet as it can help to reduce systolic blood pressure. Add a tablespoon to your breakfast cereal or mix it through soups, pasta sauce, home-baked muffin mix, stews and casseroles. You can even sprinkle it over ice cream.

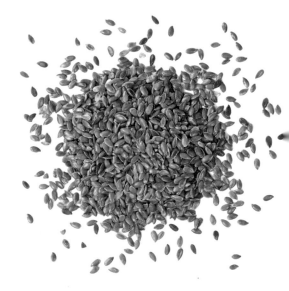

8. Shop smart

It's a tried-and-tested method of reducing bad foods in your diet – writing a shopping list before you head to the supermarket and sticking to it. If you have a list, you're more likely to avoid picking up junk food.

9. Read food labels

Just like if you're trying to lower cholesterol, read food labels so you know exactly what it is you're eating. That way, you can avoid high salt foods or foods high in saturated fats.

10. Shop the supermarket's perimeter

Most of the fresh products at the supermarket can be found around the perimeter of the shop, so shop the walls when you go. The central aisles is where you'll find packaged and processed foods, and as we are aware, fresh is best when it comes to aiding blood pressure reduction through dietary modification.

11. Drink tea instead of coffee

Drinking more than four cups of coffee a day can increase your blood pressure so find alternatives. Tea is a better option, and there have even been studies to suggest that a cup of tea can decrease systolic pressure by two points and diastolic pressure by one point. The benefits end after four cups, so perhaps stop there.

12. Swap your full-fat cafe latte for a skinny cappuccino

A large cafe latte with full cream milk contains about one third of the daily recommended fat intake for women. Add a vanilla shot and you consume the same amount of fat as eating ten rashers of bacon. Again, stick to tea, or ask for a skinny cappuccino instead. Consider a sprinkling of cinnamon instead of chocolate on top.

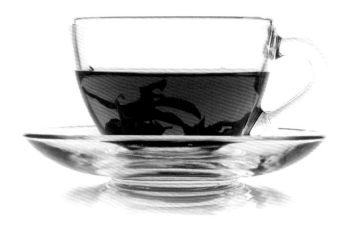

13. Be aware that some foods affect blood pressure medications

A recent Japanese study, published in the journal *Clinical Pharmacology & Therapeutics*, has found that green tea may interfere with certain blood pressure medications. Previous studies have also found that grapefruit, orange and apple juice can affect some hypertension medications by inhibiting the transporters that allow drugs to enter cells. Talk with your doctor about what should be avoided if you are being treated medically for hypertension.

14. Don't be too hard on yourself

Don't cut out all of the foods you love as it's not really sustainable and can lead to bingeing and things can quickly unravel. You can treat yourself occasionally. Perhaps slot in an extra exercise session if you do indulge to negate the effects.

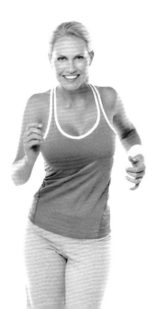

15. Eat dark chocolate instead of white and milk chocolate

When you do feel the need to indulge, make smart but indulgent choices. Unlike milk and white chocolate, dark chocolate contains flavonoids, which help to keep your arteries flexible thus preventing increases in pressure that comes with less flexible arteries. There are published studies that say small amounts of dark chocolate can lower blood pressure in older people with isolated systolic hypertension (only upper number of blood pressure reading is high). Other good sources of flavonoids, and healthier options than dark chocolate, are fruits and vegetables.

16. Snack on soy nuts

Studies have shown that eating 30 grams of soy nuts each day for two weeks can lower systolic blood pressure by an average of 10 points. Just make sure you choose an unsalted variety.

17. Gradually reduce added salt in your foods

By gradually reducing your added salt, your palette adjusts and food won't taste bland without it.

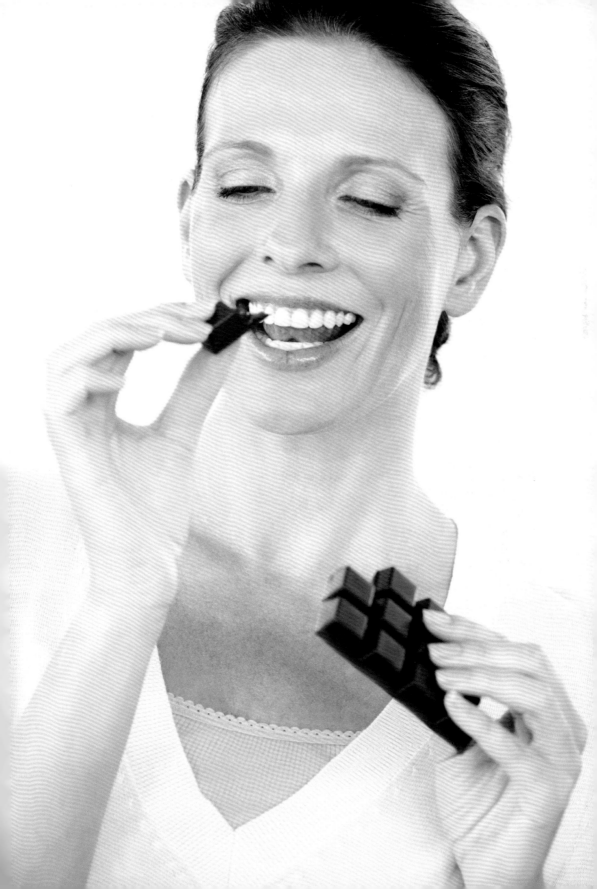

18. Flavour food with lots of pepper

When you reduce your added salt, sprinkle with a generous dose of pepper instead. It has a strong flavour and will help to retrain your taste buds to adjust to life without a lot of salt. Garlic is another alternative, or ginger, basil, lemon and other spicy flavours.

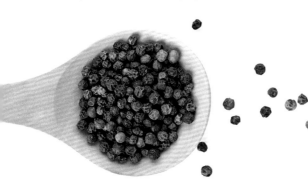

19. Limit your alcohol intake

In small amounts, alcohol can lower your blood pressure by 2-4mmHg, but that protective effect dissipates if you drink more than one standard drink each day for women and men aged over 65, and two standard drinks for men under 65. More than the recommended level can actually increase blood pressure and may interfere with blood pressure medications. Don't take up drinking alcohol if you don't already drink as there are other ways to lower blood pressure.

20. Keep track of your drinking

An alcohol diary, like your food diary, is a good way to help you to monitor your alcohol intake. If you do drink more than recommended, or are a heavy drinker, rather than suddenly eliminating alcohol, which can trigger high blood pressure for several days, taper off slowly under the supervision of your doctor.

21. Don't binge drink

Don't think you can drink all of your week's worth of safe alcohol level in one sitting. Having four or more drinks in a row can cause large and sudden blood pressure elevations.

22. Hold hands with your partner for ten minutes

We've long heard of the health benefits of a good hug but holding hands with your partner for ten minutes can keep blood pressure steady during a stressful incident.

23. Sleep with earplugs in

There have been studies that suggest noise while your sleeping can both increase blood pressure and heart rate. So consider sleeping with ear plugs, if that's safe in your household, to block out noise.

24. Drink a glass of orange juice every morning and night

Drinking a glass of orange juice twice daily has been reported in a US study to lower systolic pressure by an average of seven per cent and diastolic pressure by an average of 4.6 per cent because of the high level of potassium in oranges.

25. Ask about sleep apnoea

If there are any concerns that you may have sleep apnoea, a condition where you stop breathing many times during sleep, have it checked out as it can contribute to hypertension.

26. Ask your doctor about the use of garlic supplements

It's worth talking to your doctor about whether garlic supplements are a good option for you. It's thought that garlic counters high blood pressure because it stimulates production of the chemicals nitric oxide and hydrogen sulphide, which helps to relax blood vessels. Garlic in its raw state is healthy and contains the active ingredient allacin, but when it's cooked, allacin can be destroyed. Certain garlic supplements have a guaranteed allacin release.

27. Swap sauces

If you really feel like having a bowl of pasta for your dinner and your go-to dish has a cream-based sauce, simply swapping to a tomato-based sauce can make a difference to your overall calorie and saturated fat intakes, which can only help with your blood pressure-lowering regime.

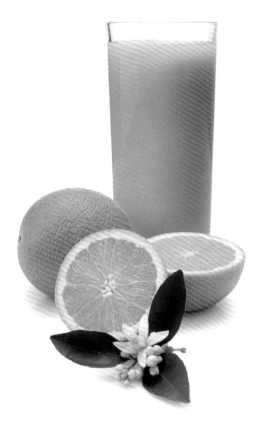

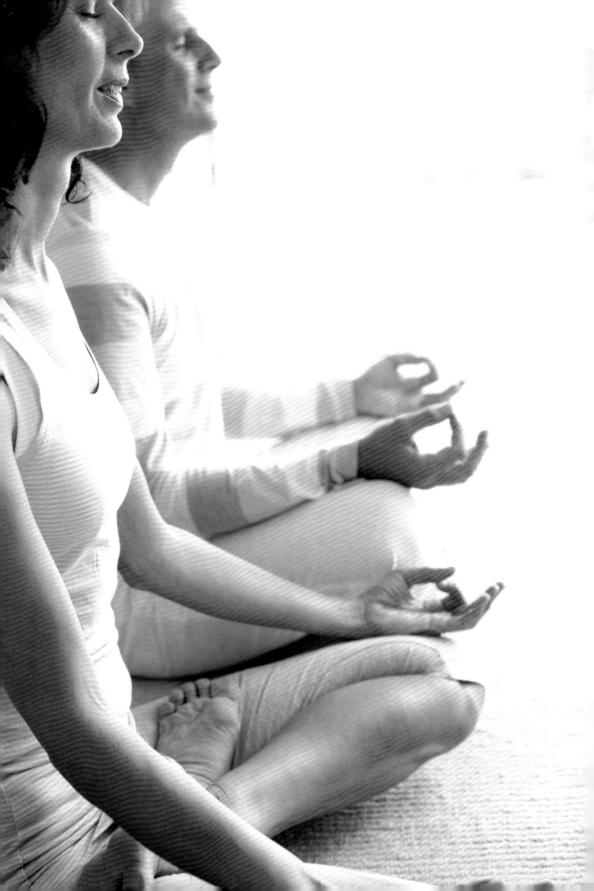

28. Make simple food substitutions

Again, making simple food swaps can help to lower your blood pressure. Instead of tossing your cooked vegetables in butter, try splashing on some lemon juice and a good sprinkling of freshly ground pepper. Eating wholegrain crisp bread instead of crackers is another wise change, as is dipping vegetable sticks in salsa or guacamole rather than eating corn chips with a cream cheese dip.

29. Work standing up when possible

If you have a desk job, try swapping sitting down at your desk with standing instead. A height adjustable desk is a great acquisition. Office workers spend about 80 per cent of their working day sitting. Researcher Professor David Dunstan of the Baker IDI Heart and Diabetes Unit says replacing four hours of sitting time with standing up, over a five-day working week, has a net gain equivalent of a brisk 45-minute walk.

30. Stop smoking

Again, like when trying to lower cholesterol, you shouldn't smoke or expose yourself to second-hand smoke. The nicotine in tobacco can raise your blood pressure by 10mmHg or more for up to an hour after smoking or inhaling other people's smoke.

31. Adopt stress management techniques

Stress and anxiety can temporarily increase blood pressure. Once you know what your stress triggers are, work at reducing them. If the stressors can't be reduced or eliminated, work on ways to help you cope with them better, including yoga, meditation, deep-breathing or get a massage.

32. Choose low salt foods

Choose foods that are labelled no-salt, low-salt or salt-reduced over full salt versions.

33. Avoid manufactured or processed foods

These types of foods, like potato chips, sausages, canned soups and packaged meals, usually have high salt contents. Avoid them when possible.

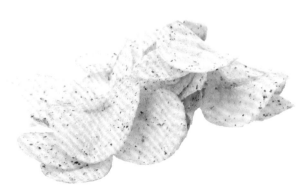

34. Drink beetroot juice

Studies show that drinking 500ml of nitrate-rich beetroot juice daily can improve heart function, lower blood pressure and increase exercise performance.

35. Take vitamin C supplements

Ask your doctor if vitamin C supplements can help you to lower your blood pressure. Researchers looked at 29 studies into the effects of vitamin C on blood pressure and the results consistently indicated that both diastolic and systolic readings were lowered after taking an average of 500milligrams per day. It is believed that vitamin C may protect levels of nitric acid, a natural compound that helps blood vessels maintain normal blood pressure.

36. Talk to your doctor about use of fish oil supplements

Studies confirm that regular consumption of fish and fish oils can lower blood pressure because of its effect on minimising atherosclerosis and the reduction of triglyceride levels. Talk to your doctor about fish oil supplementation because the effects appear to be dose-dependent.

37. Discuss vitamin D supplementation closely with your doctor

There is debate around the efficacy of vitamin D supplementation on lowering blood pressure. A Harvard study found that women with low vitamin D levels were at increased risk of hypertension, whereas other studies indicate there is little evidence that vitamin D reduces blood pressure. After discussing with your doctor, make an informed choice together.

38. Look into the use of CoQ10

In consultation with your doctor, consider supplementing with coenzyme Q10. Some researchers suggest that up to a third of people with hypertension have low levels of this coenzyme. It is believed that CoQ10 may lower blood pressure by reducing free radical damage inside arteries. Talk with your doctor into its possible use for you.

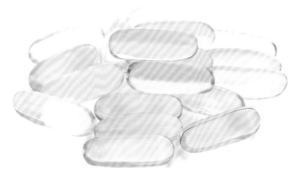

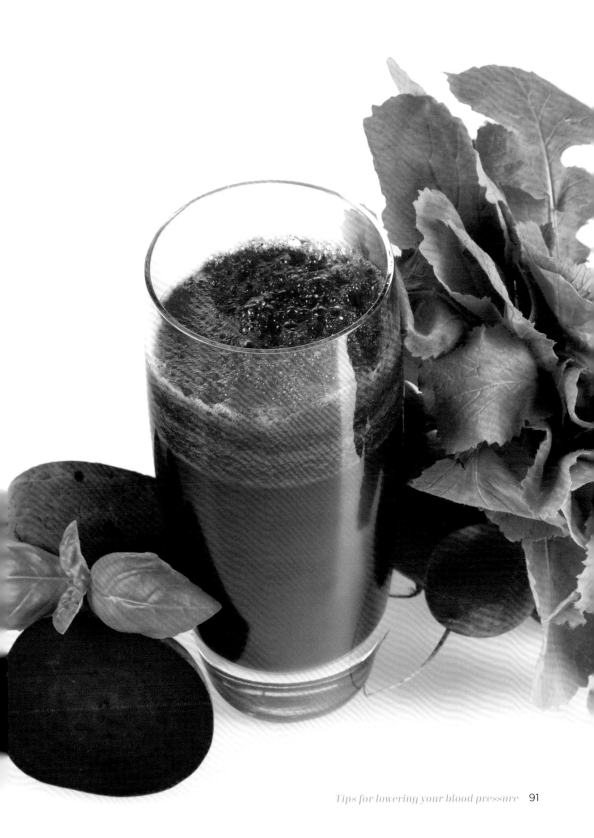

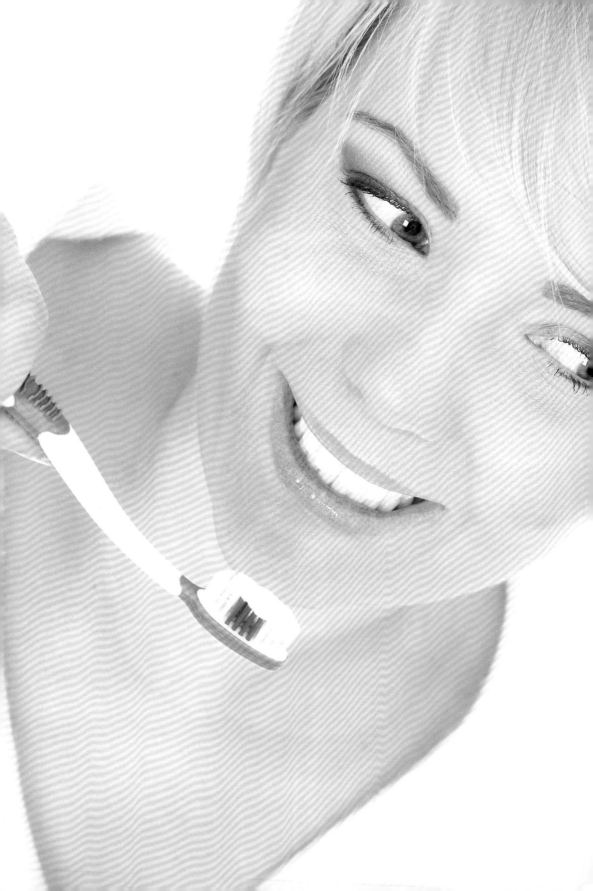

39. Have a laugh

Laughing is basically like aerobics for your insides. When we laugh, as many as 400 of our muscles move, and after hearty laughter, heart rate and blood pressure drop to a level lower than the initial resting rate. Endorphins, our feel-good hormones, are also released with laughter and the stress hormones adrenaline and cortisol are reduced. It may only offer a temporary blood pressure drop but it's good fun doing it.

40. Sprinkle linseeds on breakfast

A study found that adding four tablespoons of linseed, split between breakfast and a later meal, reduced blood pressure in postmenopausal women with a history of heart disease. Linseeds are nutrient-rich and high in fibre.

41. Brush and floss your teeth twice a day

For more than 20 years, dental health has been linked to heart disease. It is thought that there is a connection between serious gum disease and atherosclerosis, the build-up of fatty deposits on the artery walls. While conclusive evidence is still yet to be found, the American Heart Association has said that a link is 'biologically plausible. So, brush and floss your teeth twice a day just to be on the safe side.

42. Dressing on the side

Always ask for your salad dressing or sauces to be in a separate vessel when you order food at a cafe or restaurant. That way, you can control how much dressing or sauce (traditionally high in hidden sugars) you consume.

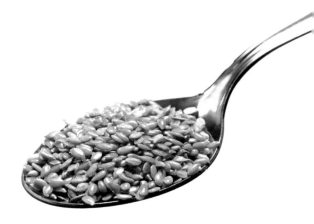

43. Invest in some good cookware

There are some amazing non-stick frying pans available on the market that mean you don't have to use oil to grease your pan before cooking, and silicon bakeware often means you don't have to grease with butter before baking. Invest in good cookware so you don't use unnecessary fats during cooking.

44. Cut off the fat

When you buy bacon, buy the rindless variety, and when you buy a steak, choose lean cuts or chop off the fat before cooking. Most supermarkets and some butchers have a heart smart or premium grade mince option. It's a far better alternative than the regular three-star option. Add extra herbs or garlic to your healthier mince to give added flavour.

45. Ask your doctor about the DASH diet

The DASH diet (Dietary Approaches to Stop Hypertension) is recognised by leading health authorities, including the American Heart Association and The American College of Cardiology, as being a healthy and safe diet to follow because of its emphasis on fruits, vegetables, whole grains, low-fat dairy, poultry, fish and nuts. It can also help to lower both blood pressure and cholesterol. Talk to your doctor about the benefits of following the DASH diet plan.

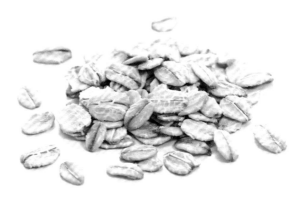

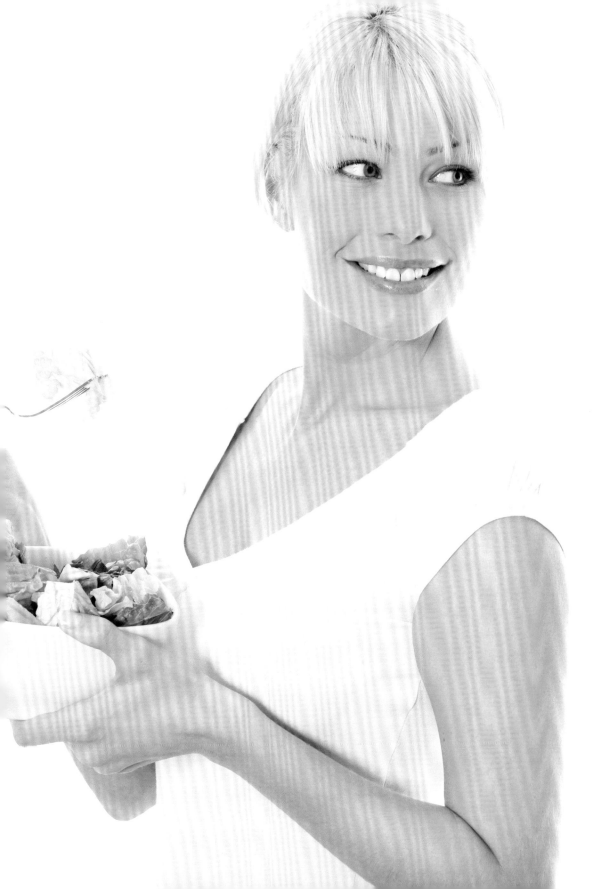

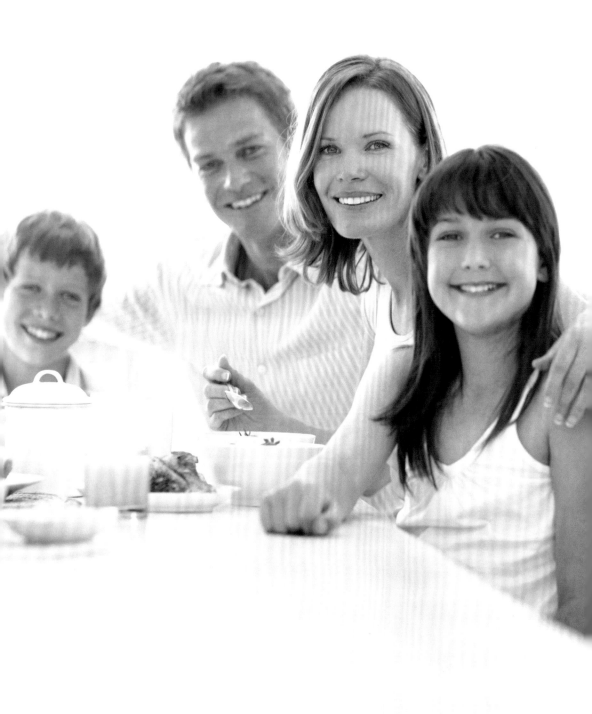

Recipes to help with blood pressure and cholesterol management

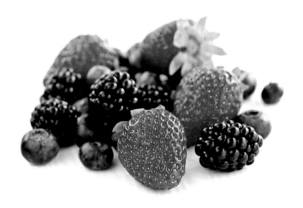

Breakfast/ Brunch

Apple-berry compote with natural yoghurt

Ingredients
4 medium-sized apples peeled and cored
(you can use apples that are past their best)
100ml freshly squeezed orange juice
Pinch of cinnamon
1 cup of berries (fresh are best but frozen
are good too)
1/2 cup natural yoghurt
1 tablespoon flaxseeds
Serves 4

Method
Chop your apples into chunks, then put them
in a heavy-based pan with the orange juice
and cinnamon. Cook over a low heat for
about 10 minutes or until just tender. Add
your berries until they're warm, then serve
immediately with a dollop of natural or low-fat
yoghurt and a sprinkle of flaxseeds.

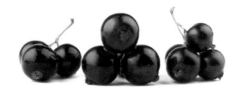

Granola

Ingredients
2 tablespoons grape seed oil
2 cups rolled oats
1/4 cup sesame seeds
1/4 cup sunflower seeds
1/2 cup slivered almonds
1/2 cup shredded coconut
1/2 cup honey
1 tablespoon vanilla extract
1 tablespoon orange zest
1 tablespoon cinnamon

Method
Toss the oats, seeds, nuts and coconut together
in a large bowl. In another bowl, combine
the grape seed oil, honey, vanilla extract and
orange zest. Add the dry ingredients to the
runny mixture and give everything a good
mix. Tip the mixture onto a baking sheet lined
with baking paper and sprinkle the cinnamon
over the top. Place in a pre-heated 200 degree
celsius oven and bake for about 20 minutes.
Check the granola occasionally to ensure the
mixture doesn't catch. Once baked, remove
from oven and slide the baking paper onto a
wire rack to allow the mixture to cool. Once
cooled, break up into clusters and keep in an
airtight container in the freezer. The granola
stays beautifully crunchy and can be served
straight out of the freezer. Serve with a splash
of low-fat milk and blueberries. One serve is
about 5 tablespoons of granola.

Kicking egg white omelette

Ingredients
4 egg whites
1/4 diced red capsicum
1/4 diced yellow capsicum
1/4 cup diced red onion
1 red chili (deseeded if you don't like too much kick)
Fresh basil leaves
1 tablespoon extra-virgin olive oil
Serves 1

Method
Heat oil over a medium heat in a small frying pan. Sauté your onions and capsicum until soft, before adding your chili and cooking for a further 45 seconds or so. Pour the egg whites over the mixture, then add some fresh basil leaves. As the eggs begin to set, gently lift the sides of the omelette so the uncooked egg slides underneath. Repeat this process until the omelette is set, then flip the omelette to cook on the other side for just a few seconds with a good sprinkle of freshly cracked pepper. Fold your omelette over and remove from the pan onto your serving plate. A sprinkle of low-fat cheese can be added for extra flavour.

Full-cooked brekkie

Ingredients
2 eggs
Splash of skim milk
Splash of extra virgin olive oil
1 rasher of lean bacon
1 cup of spinach
1 clove of garlic
1 tomato sliced
6 mushrooms sliced
1 slice of multigrain toast
Cracked pepper

Method
Changing your cooking methods helps to make this a healthier version of a full-cooked English breakfast. Firstly, mix your eggs with a splash of skim milk, then pop them into a microwave-safe dish and cook for 30 seconds at a time until they're scrambled and cooked to your liking. Grill your tomatoes, mushrooms and bacon rasher to eliminate the need for fat, and add a crack of pepper to each. Steam your spinach in the microwave, or add a splash of water to a pan before adding your spinach and wilting it on the stove. Grill the bread, then rub your garlic clove over the top to add flavour. You can spread your toast with a little monounsaturated rich, olive oil-based spread or one of the cholesterol-lowering spreads available at most supermarkets.

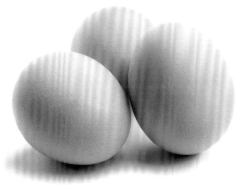

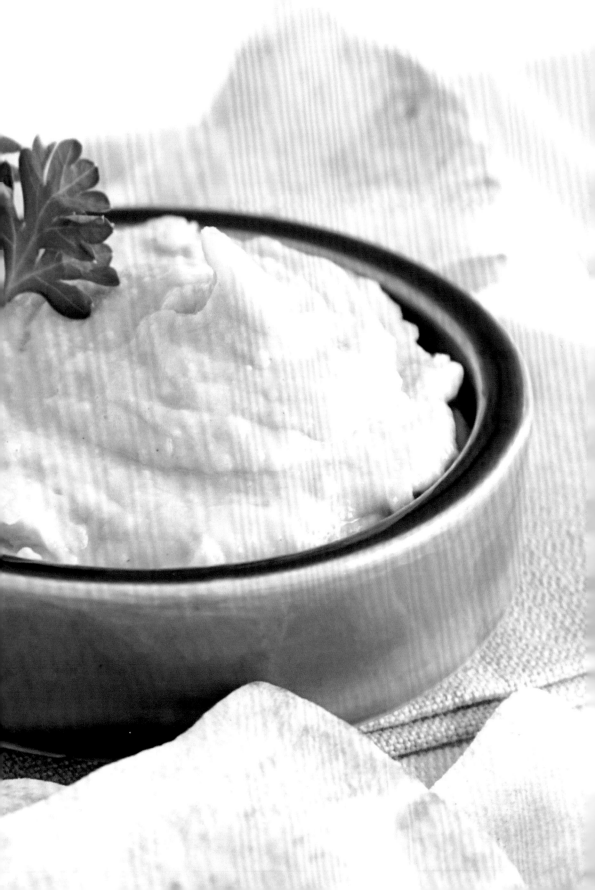

Lunch

Hummus on pitta

Ingredients

1 can of chickpeas
2/3 pot of set low-fat plain yoghurt
1-2 cloves of garlic
Pinch of paprika
Pinch or ground cumin
1 tablespoon flaxseeds
Juice of half a lemon
2 wholegrain pitta breads
1 tomato
Sliced cucumber
Serves 2

Method

Drain and rinse the chickpeas, then add to a blender with the yoghurt, garlic, spices, flaxseeds and lemon juice. Blend until smooth. Place your pitta bread in a dry frying pan for 30 seconds on each side, or until it starts to go crunchy. Place your hummus, sliced tomato and cucumber on top of your pitta bread to serve.

Leek and asparagus frittata

Ingredients

1 tablespoon extra-virgin olive oil
1 bunch of asparagus, trimmed and chopped into 3cm pieces. Keep the stems and tips separate
1 leek, washed well and sliced
1 tablespoon wholemeal flour
3 eggs lightly beaten
Bunch of fresh basil
Baby rocket, to serve
Balsamic vinegar, to serve

Method

Heat the oil in a non-stick frying pan over a medium heat. Cook the leeks for about 5 minutes until soft, stirring occasionally. Add the asparagus stems and cook for 3 minutes, then add the asparagus tips and cook for a further two minutes. Mix the flour with a teaspoon of water and enough of the lightly beaten egg to make a runny paste. Add the flour paste to the remaining egg. Add the basil to the mixture, give it a little mix and then add to the pan, stirring gently to cover the vegetables. When it's almost set, lower the heat and cover the pan with foil and cook for a further 2-3 minutes until set. Serve with the rocket and balsamic.

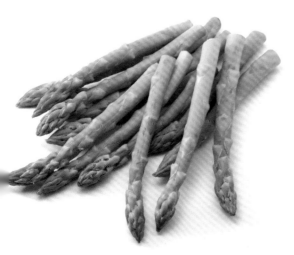

Homemade baked beans on multi

Ingredients

400g can of mixed beans, drained
2 cloves garlic, finely sliced
1/2 red onion
Can of reduced-salt tinned tomatoes
1 tablespoon of Worcestershire sauce
1 teaspoon of brown sugar
Multigrain bread
1 teaspoon extra virgin olive oil

Method

Heat oil in saucepan over a medium heat. Add the onion and garlic and cook for 1-2 minutes. Add the tomatoes, sugar and Worcestershire sauce and cook for another 2-3 minutes, before adding the beans and cooking for a further 2 minutes. Toast your bread and add a scrape of monounsaturated, olive oil-based spread to it, or cholesterol-lowering spread available from most supermarkets, if you don't like toast with no spread. Serve the beans on top.

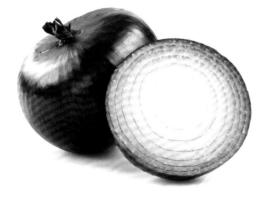

Chicken, avocado and tomato wrap

Ingredients

450g chicken breast, skinless with all fat removed, thinly sliced
1 tablespoon extra-virgin olive oil
1 large red onion, thinly sliced
1 red capsicum, thinly sliced
1 yellow capsicum, thinly sliced
Pinch (about 1/8 of a teaspoon) of paprika
Pinch mild chili powder
2 pinches of cumin
2 pinches of dried oregano
4 wholemeal or multigrain tortillas
1/2 iceberg lettuce, finely shredded
Avocado
1 small red onion, finely chopped
425g sweet tomatoes
2 garlic cloves, crushed
Large handful of fresh coriander leaves, chopped
Freshly cracked black pepper
Serves 4

Method

Combine chopped tomatoes, red onion, garlic and coriander and a crack of black pepper in a bowl, and cover and chill for 30 minutes for the flavours in the salsa to develop. Heat the oil in a wok and stir fry the onion and capsicum for 3-4 minutes. Add the thinly sliced chicken pieces, cumin, paprika, chilli and oregano, and cook for another five minutes until the chicken is cooked. Meanwhile, wrap the tortillas in foil and put in a warm oven to heat through. Place the chicken mixture, a spoonful of salsa and a tablespoon of lightly smashed avocado on the tortilla and serve.

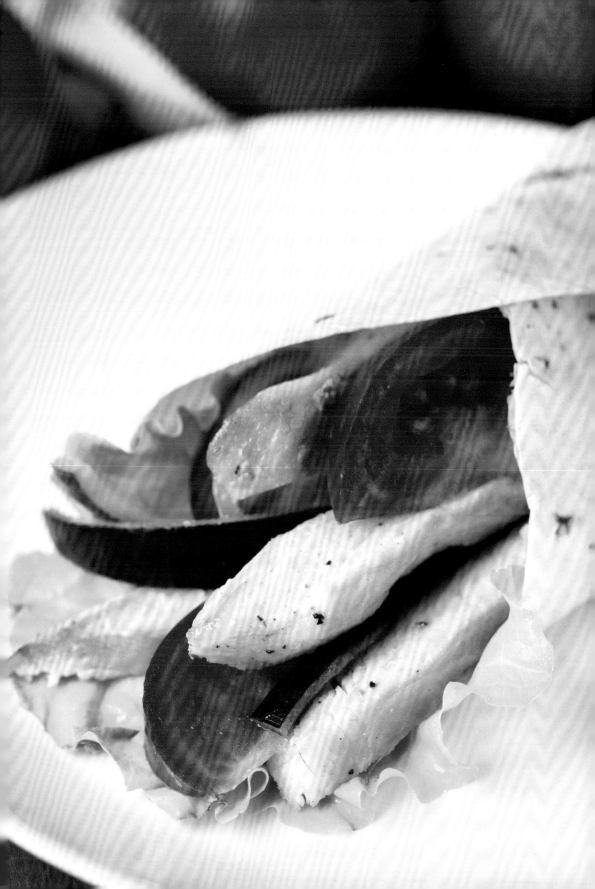

Parsnip and apple soup

Ingredients

600g parsnips, with woody centres removed, cut into 2cm pieces
600g apples (Granny Smiths, Bramleys, even Pink Lady), peeled and cut into chunks
2 medium-sized onions, chopped
2 garlic cloves, crushed
25g salt-reduced butter
1 tbsp sunflower oil
1 litre salt-reduced chicken or vegetable stock
150ml reduced fat milk
Freshly ground black pepper

Method

Melt butter in the oil in a large saucepan and gently fry the onions and parsnips for about 15 minutes or until the onions are soft and translucent. Add the apples and crushed garlic and cook for another two minutes, stirring regularly (at this point you could add spices like ground cumin, coriander and/or ginger for another dimension). Add the stock and bring to the boil before reducing the heat and simmering for about 20 minutes or until the parsnips are super soft. Season with the pepper then blend in a food processor until smooth. Stir through the milk to add a little creaminess.

Italian mixed bean soup

Ingredients

2 onions
2 carrots
2 stalks of celery
1 can red kidney beans
1 can chickpeas
1 can borlotti beans
1 can crushed tomatoes
450ml salt-reduced chicken stock
1 clove garlic
1/2 cup fresh basil
2 tbsp fresh oregano
1 tbsp olive oil
1/2 cup parmesan cheese, freshly grated
Crack of black pepper

Method

Heat the oil in a large saucepan over a medium heat. Gently fry the onions, carrots and celery until soft. Add the crouched garlic and cook for another minute before adding the stock, tomatoes, basil and oregano. Bring to the boil, then reduce the heat and simmer, partially-covered, for another 10 minutes. After rinsing the canned beans, stir them through the soup and cook for another 10 minutes. Remove from heat. Take about 2 cups of the mixture out and, using a hand blender, give it a bit of a blitz until it's a coarse puree. Return the coarse puree to the remaining soup and serve with a sprinkle of parmesan cheese and a crack of black pepper.

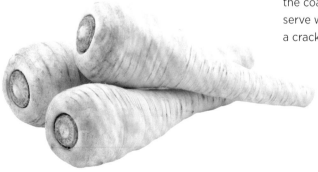

Baked sweet potato

Ingredients

2 sweet potatoes
1 red chili, finely chopped (deseeded if you don't like things too hot)
4 spring onions, finely chopped
2 tablespoons of low fat cream cheese
Splash of extra virgin olive oil

Method

Heat oven to 180 degrees. Prick your sweet potatoes and place them on a baking tray lined with baking paper. Put them in the oven for about an hour, or until they are nice and soft. Remove from the oven and slice down the middle lengthways. Scatter the spring onions inside the opening, then add a dollop of low fat cream cheese. Sprinkle the chopped chili over and a splash of olive oil to serve.

Three pea salad

Ingredients

200g sugar snap peas
200g snow peas
200g frozen peas
25g goat's cheese crumbled (optional)
1/4 cup flaked almonds toasted
1/3 cup fresh mint finely chopped

Dressing

2 tablespoons extra virgin olive oil
1 tablespoon white wine vinegar
1 teaspoon sugar
Serves four

Method

Blanch all pea varieties in boiling water for about 60 seconds, then plunge them into ice cold water to stop the cooking process. Drain well. Shake up the mint, olive oil, vinegar and sugar in a screw top jar. Toss the peas through the dressing and then top with the toasted flaked almonds and a sprinkle of goat's cheese.

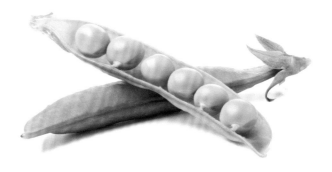

Kedgeree

Ingredients

200g brown rice
400g smoked salmon or smoked haddock, cooked
4 medium eggs, hard boiled
1 level teaspoon cumin seeds
2 level teaspoons curry powder
2 level teaspoons grated root ginger
1 clove garlic, crushed,
8 spring onions, finely chopped
1 red chilli, finely sliced and deseeded
100g frozen peas
2 tablespoons fresh parsley
Splash of canola oil
Freshly cracked black pepper

Method

Cook your brown rice in simmering water for about 30 minutes or until al dente. In a large frying pan, cover your fish with water and let it simmer gently for about five minutes. Remove any skin and bones, then flake the fish into chunks. Boil your eggs, then cool in cold water and remove their shells. In a wok, add a splash of canola oil and gently fry the spring onions, garlic, chili and ginger for about 5 minutes. Add the well-drained rice to the pan with the curry, cumin and peas and cook for a further two minutes. Gently stir through the parsley and fish. Season with a good crack of freshly ground black pepper and serve topped with quartered boiled eggs and another sprinkling of fresh parsley.

Artichoke and bean sandwich

Ingredients

1 can of haricot/cannellini beans
Splash of basil-infused olive oil (or pummel fresh basil leaves with a splash of olive oil in a mortar and pestle)
1 artichoke heart (from your deli or even a jar)
6 semi-sundried/blushed tomatoes, drained of oil
Slices of red onion
Slice of multigrain/granary bread

Method

Toast your bread. Drain the beans and mash with the back of a fork with a little basil oil. Spoon the beans over the toast and top with the artichoke hearts, sundried tomatoes and a few slices of red onion.

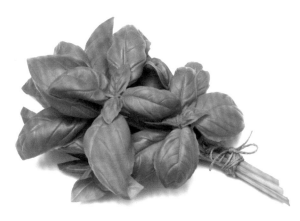

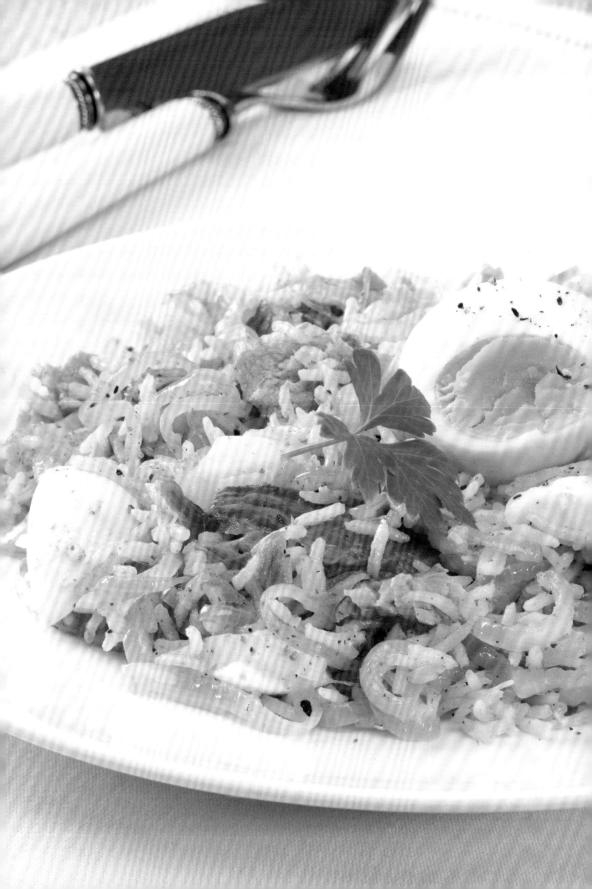

Sardine open sarnie

Ingredients

1 clove of garlic, cut in half
1 tomato
Rocket
Quality can of sardines (fresh sardines can be hard to come by and rot quickly but if you're able to, fresh is best)
Thick slice of multigrain/granary bread

Method

Toast your bread and rub the cut side of the garlic clove over the surface. Cut your tomato in half and squeeze it over the toast, then rub the flesh over the toast's surface. Place your sardines on top and then pile your rocket on.

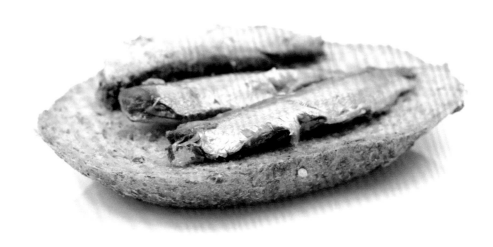

Dinner

Spice-crusted salmon with asian slaw

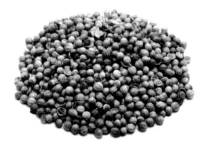

Ingredients
4 salmon fillets, skin on
1 teaspoon fennel seeds
1 teaspoon coriander seeds
1 teaspoon yellow mustard seeds
Freshly ground black pepper
3 tablespoons canola oil
1/4 white cabbage
1/4 red cabbage
1 large carrot
1 green apple
1/2 red capsicum
Handful of bean sprouts
1 tablespoon lime juice
1 tablespoon fresh coriander, finely chopped
2 tablespoons sunflower oil
1/2 teaspoon sesame oil
1 teaspoon grated fresh ginger

Method
Toast the fennel, coriander and mustard seeds in a dry pan on a low heat for about 8 minutes or until you start to smell the fragrant aromas. Crush the seeds in a mortar and pestle and add a little freshly ground black pepper. Slash the salmon skins three times, then lay the fish on the spice mix, skin side up, so the spices cover the underside of the fish. Ideally, leave for about two hours; 20 minutes at the very least. Shred the cabbages, capsicum, carrot and apple in a food processor, then add the bean sprouts. Whisk together the lime juice, sunflower and sesame oils, ginger and coriander and toss over the Asian slaw mix. Rub the salmon with the canola oil and fry skin side down on a medium heat, pressing down lightly. Try not to move the salmon for five or six minutes so the skin goes nice and crispy. When the edges are golden, turn the fish over and cup for a further 1 minute. Serve the salmon on the side of the Asian slaw.

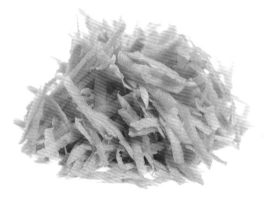

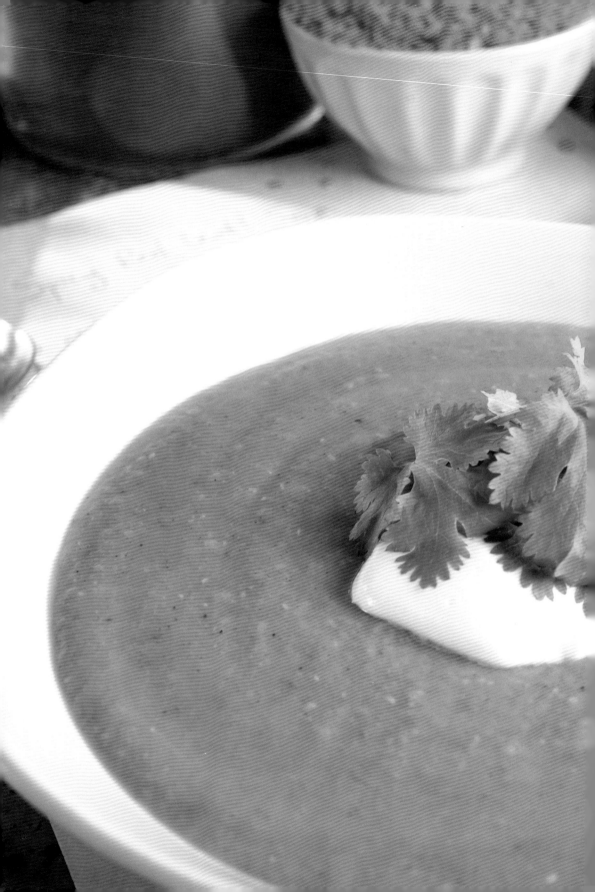

Barbecued salmon with beetroot and quinoa salad

Ingredients

2 beetroots, peeled and quartered
2 carrots
1 green apple or pear
1 cup of quinoa
2 handfuls of fresh coriander
Juice of 1/2 lemon
Half an avocado
Handful of walnuts
2 handfuls of rocket
2 salmon fillets
Splash of extra virgin olive oil

Method

In a food processor, chop the beetroots, carrots, apple or pear and coriander. Toss through the quinoa, then top it on the bed of rocket. Squeeze your lemon juice over and sprinkle with walnuts. Rub a little olive oil over your salmon and add a good crack of black pepper, then place it skin side up first on your barbecue plate. Flip it over after about three minutes and cook for another five minutes or so until cooked to your liking. Squeeze a little lemon over the top and serve with the salad.

Cumin, carrot and red lentil soup

Ingredients

1.2 litres of sale-reduced vegetable stock
1 cup of red lentils
1 large onion, chopped
3 large carrots, thick slices
2 large vine-ripened tomatoes, chopped up
1 red chilli
1 green chilli
2 cloves of garlic, roughly chopped
2 tablespoons of salt-reduced tomato puree
1 teaspoon cumin
1 teaspoon curry powder
1 teaspoon coriander
1 tablespoon olive oil

Method

Over low-medium heat, warm the olive oil in a large saucepan, then add the garlic, onion and chilli. Cook gently until the onion is soft and transparent. Add the spices, tomato and tomato puree and fry for a further five minutes, stirring regularly. Add the rest of the ingredients and stir well, then put a lid on your pan and let the soup simmer away for about 25 minutes or until the lentils are soft. Blend the soup in a blender or in the pan with a stick blender until it's the consistency you like.

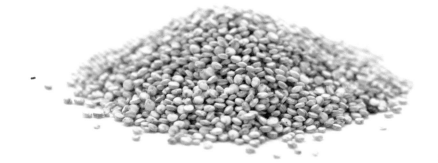

Tuna steak stir-fry

Ingredients

2 tuna steaks
1 large onion, finely chopped
1 large carrot, finely sliced
Handful of snow peas/mange tout
1/2 red capsicum, finely sliced
1 clove of garlic
2 tablespoons fresh coriander, crushed
1/2 teaspoon ground ginger
1 tablespoon sesame oil
2 tablespoons low salt soy sauce
200g fine rice noodles

Method

Chop the tuna into thick slices and marinate in the lime juice mixed with the crushed coriander leaves for about two hours. Cook your rice noodles as instructed on the packet, then heat your oil in a large wok. Add the onion and carrot and fry for a couple of minutes before adding the garlic, capsicum and snow peas and cooking for a minute longer. Pour over the soy sauce, then add the ginger and marinated tuna along with the lime and coriander marinade. Cook until tuna is cooked through. Add a final scattering on fresh coriander just before serving over the drained noodles.

Barramundi on a salsa bed

Ingredients

4 pieces of barramundi
1 tablespoon flour
1-2 tablespoons extra-virgin olive oil
Crack of freshly ground pepper
1 mango, finely diced
1 avocado, finely diced
1 small red onion, finely diced
1 bunch of asparagus

Method

Coat your fish in the peppered flour, then shake off the excess. Pan fry your barramundi in the oil over a medium heat. Remove the fibrous end of your asparagus and then cook the spears in a griddle pan with a little oil and a crack of pepper. Serve your fish on top of the mango, avocado and red onion salsa mix with the asparagus on the side.

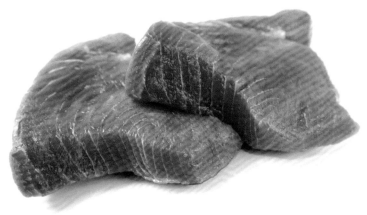

Lamb koftas with cranberry and pearl couscous tabouli

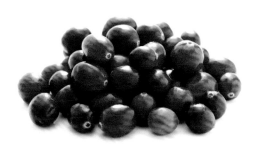

Ingredients

500g lean lamb mince
2 small tomatoes, diced
2 teaspoons pomegranate molasses
4 large garlic cloves, chopped.
1.5 tablespoons harissa spice blend
1.5 tablespoons extra virgin olive oil
1 cup eggplant dip
2 wholemeal or multigrain flat breads
1/2 cup pearl couscous
1/2 cup water
1 teaspoon of cholesterol-lowering /olive oil-based spread
4 spring onions
2 cups parsley leaves
1 cup mint leaves
2 garlic cloves
4 medium tomatoes
1/2 cup dried cranberries
1 tablespoon lemon juice
Serves 4

Method

Put mince, tomatoes, pomegranate molasses, garlic and harissa into a large bowl and mix well. Divide the mix into two and then each half into two and shape the mix into four sausage shapes. On a medium-heat barbecue, grill the koftas, turning frequently, and brushing with the olive oil. After between 10 and 15 minutes, remove from heat but wrap your koftas in foil to keep them warm. Half you flatbreads and warm them through on the barbecue. Cook your pearl couscous according to packet instructions, using the cholesterol-lowering margarine instead of butter if required. Place the herbs, onions and garlic into a little food processor and chop finely, before stirring it, and the tomatoes, cranberries and lemon, into the couscous. Place your kofta, a little eggplant dip and couscous tabouli onto the flatbread and wrap to serve.

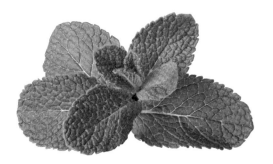

Spaghetti Bolognese

Ingredients

500g lean/heart smart beef mince (or use half pork mince and half beef mince)
1-2 tablespoons canola oil
1 large onion, finely diced
1 medium zucchini/courgette, grated
2 large carrots, grated
10 button mushrooms, halved
3 cloves of garlic
Can of salt reduced tomatoes
4 tablespoons salt reduced tomato puree
1/2 tablespoon dried oregano
1/2 tablespoon dried parsley
1/2 tablespoon dried basil
2 tablespoons Worcestershire sauce
400g wholemeal spaghetti

Method

Fry onions in the canola oil over a medium heat in a large pot. Add the mince and cook until it's browned, then add the garlic. Place the grated vegetables into the mix and give them a good toss around for about three minutes before adding the tin of tomatoes and puree. Next, add the herbs and Worcester sauce and simmer for about 20 minutes. Cook pasta according to the packet instructions, then mix the pasta through the meaty sauce.

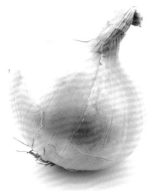

Kidney bean and rice burger

Ingredients

3/4 cup brown rice, cooked
Can of red kidney beans
1/2 cup onion, finely chopped,
1/4 cup celery, finely chopped
1/4 cup wholegrain breadcrumbs
2 tablespoons fresh coriander, finely chopped
1 clove garlic, minced
1/2 teaspoon dried oregano
1/2 teaspoon cumin
1/2 teaspoon freshly ground black pepper
4 multigrain rolls, split and toasted
Handful of rocket
1 tomato, sliced
1/2 red onion, finely sliced
2 tablespoons light mayonnaise
1/2 tablespoon flaxseeds
Serves 4

Method

Use a potato masher or the back of a fork to coarsely mash the kidney beans. Add the onions, celery, breadcrumbs, coriander, garlic, spices and pepper to the mashed beans and stir through, then stir in the cooked rice. Halve the mix, then halve each half to make four equally-sized patties, about 2cm thick. Add the patties to a pre-heated griddle pan over medium heat. Cook for 5-6 minutes each side or until the patties are heated through. Place the burgers on your toasted buns and mix the flaxseeds through the mayo. Top your burgers with a smear of mayo, then add the tomato, red onion and rocket.

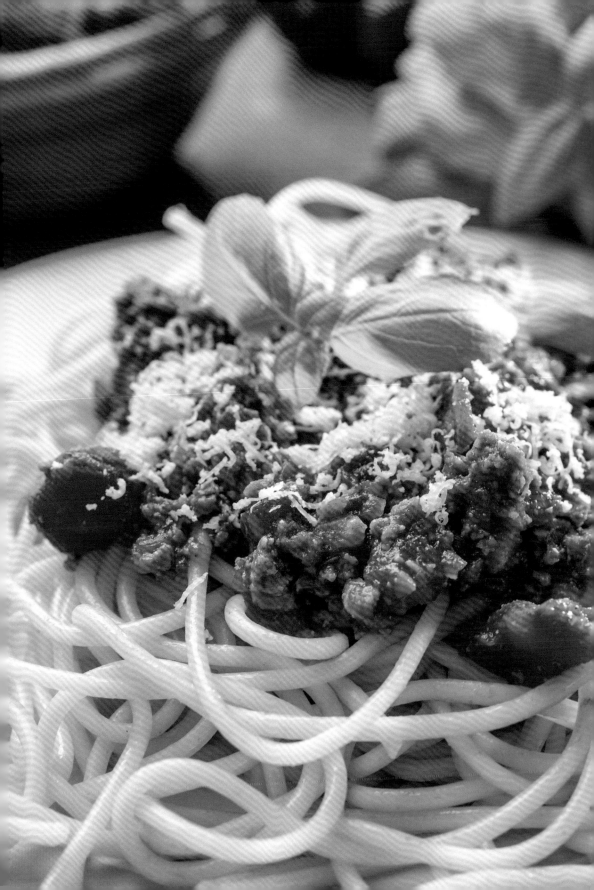

Kid's Dinner

Chicken nuggets

Ingredients
2 chicken breasts, skin off
1/2 cup buttermilk
3 cups corn flakes, crushed

Method
Chop chicken into bite-sized pieces and put in a bowl. Pour over the buttermilk and cover, then refrigerate for at least 20 minutes (but ideally a couple of hours). Place crushed corn flakes into a zip-lock bag. Drag each piece of chicken across the side of your bowl to remove excess buttermilk, then add to corn flakes and toss your nuggets around until well coated. Add to the corn flake bag in batches of no more than 6 so the mixture doesn't go mushy. Once covered, place on a lined baking sheet and bake in a pre-heated 180 degree Celsius oven.

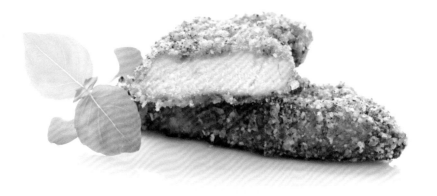

Dessert

Roasted pears with cinnamon

Ingredients

4 pears
1 tablespoon caster sugar
1 teaspoon cinnamon
Extra light olive oil spray
Natural low fat yoghurt
Extra cinnamon for sprinkling

Method

Peel and core your pears, then cut them into quarters lengthways and put in a baking dish lined with baking paper. Spray your pears with a little of the olive oil spray. Mix the caster sugar and teaspoon of cinnamon together and sprinkle over the pears. Toss them well so they are coated with the sugary mix. Roast for about 20 minutes in an oven pre-heated to 180C or until the pears are golden and tender. Add a dollop of natural low fat yoghurt and another sprinkling of cinnamon. You can add a few blanched almonds or pecans for added texture.

Plum and apple crumble

Ingredients

6 ripe plums
3 large sweet apples
125g wholemeal flour
50g soft brown sugar
50g slivered almonds
50g cholesterol-lowering olive oil-based spread
1 teaspoon cinnamon

Method

Heat your oven to 190C, then wash and core your apples and cut them into eighths, keeping the skin on. Wash and de-stone the plums, then press the apples and plums into an oven bake dish. Sprinkle with cinnamon, then rub the margarine spread in the flour until it looks like breadcrumbs. Add the almonds and brown sugar to this mix, then top the fruit mixture. Bake for between 20 and 25 minutes or until the fruit is soft and the top is golden.

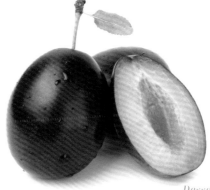

Chocolate pecan meringue cookies

Ingredients

1/3 cup of pecans or walnuts
1/2 cup icing sugar, plus little extra for sprinkling
1 tablespoon best quality cocoa powder
1/4 teaspoon cinnamon
2 large egg whites

Method

Preheat the oven to 150C and take two baking paper-lined baking trays. In a saucepan, dry toast the pecans, stirring frequently, until they become fragrant and crisp, then, once cooled, coarsely chop them. Sift the icing sugar, cinnamon and cocoa powder, then in a large, clean bowl, beat the egg whites until they form stiff peaks. Gently fold in the chocolatey mix with a spatula and then gently fold through the nuts. Being very gentle, drop large teaspoons of the mixture onto the trays and bake for about 20 minutes until set. Remove the biscuits from their trays and allow them to cool on a wire rack. Dust with icing

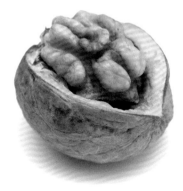

Yummy chocolate mousse

Ingredients

85g 70% dark chocolate
1tbsp cocoa powder
2 egg whites
1 tbsp instant coffee granules
1/2 tsp vanilla extract
50g full-fat Greek yoghurt
Raspberries to decorate

Method

Half-fill a medium saucepan with water and heat it until it's simmering. Finely chop up the chocolate and put it into a large bowl that can sit on top of the pan of simmering water. Mix together 2 tablespoons of cold water with the cocoa powder, coffee and vanilla, then pour over the chocolate. Put the bowl on top of the pan of simmering water, give it a little stir, then take off the heat. Keep the bowl over the simmering water and stir it occasionally until it's melted. Once melted, add 2 tablespoons of boiling water to the chocolate to thin it down, then leave it to cool slightly. Meanwhile, whisk your egg whites to soft peaks then whisk in the sugar until the mixture is glossy and thick. Beat the yoghurt through the cooled chocolate, then carefully fold about one third of the egg whites into the chocolate mix with a large metal spoon. Gently fold through the remaining egg whites. Don't over mix or you'll knock the air out of the mixture and lose volume. Divide the mixture into four ramekins and pop in the fridge for a couple of hours, or overnight. Decorate with a few raspberries, then dust with a little extra cocoa powder. Even though Greek yoghurt is quite high in fat, the other modifications make this recipe a better alternative to your traditional chocolate mousse.

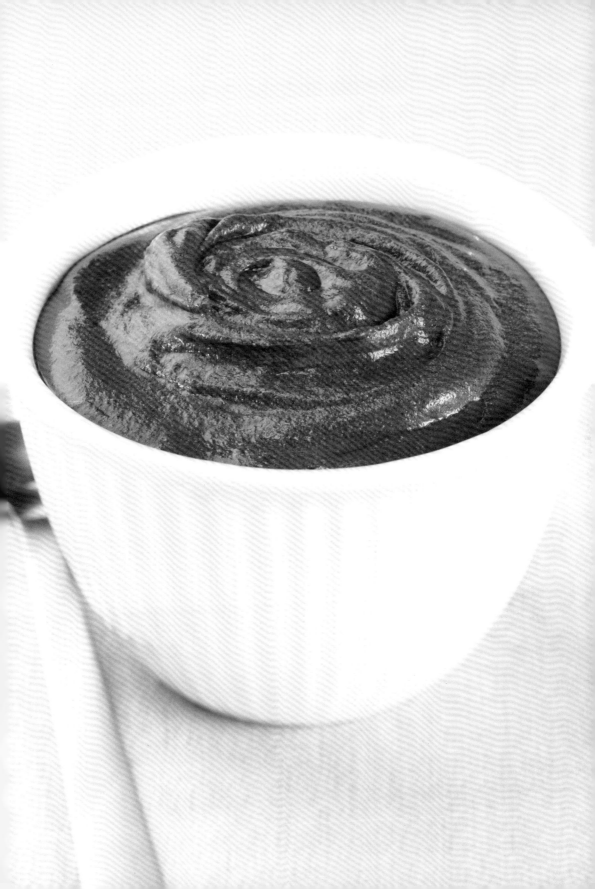

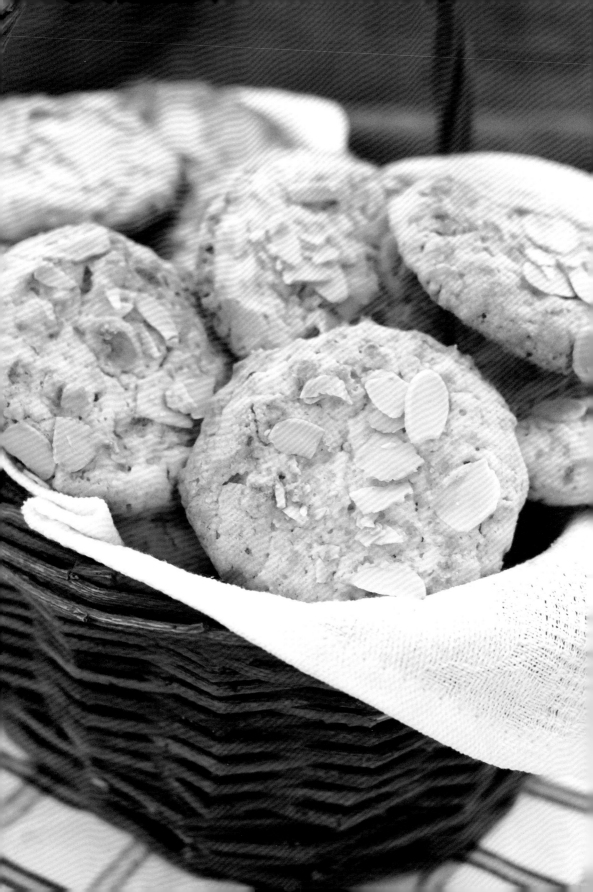

Nutty oat bikkies

Ingredients

3 teaspoons of cholesterol-lowering spread
1/4 cup wholegrain oats
1 cup flaked almonds
1 teaspoon honey
1/2 cup caster sugar
1 egg white
For topping
1/4 cup flaked almonds
1/3 cup pistachio kernels
1/2 teaspoon icing sugar

Method

Melt margarine and honey in a microwave on low power for about 30 seconds. In a food processor bowl, put the oats, almonds and sugar and process until the mixture is fine in texture. Then, with the mixer still running, pour in the egg white and the honey mixture and continue to process for another 30 seconds or so until the mixture is a smooth paste. Cover the mix and refrigerate for about an hour. Preheat your oven to 150C. Chop the almond flakes and pistachios for the topping and mix them together well. Take your refrigerated mixture and shape it into about 16 small balls. Roll the balls through the almond pistachio mix and press the nuts firmly into the mixture. Place on a lined baking tray and bake for about 20 minutes or until they're lightly browned. Cool on the tray, then serve them with a light sprinkling of the icing sugar over the top.

Cheat's Red Velvet Cupcake

Ingredients

1 cup beetroot, no salt added and pureed
1 cup egg whites
1 cup wholemeal flour
3/4 cup sugar
1/2 cup ground almonds
2 teaspoons cocoa powder
2 teaspoons baking powder
1/3 cup buttermilk
Pinch of salt
Makes 24

Method

Pre-heat your oven to 175 degrees. Beat together the egg whites and sugar with a mixer for about 2 minutes, then stir through the pureed beetroot and buttermilk. Meanwhile, combine the baking powder, flour, almonds, cocoa powder and salt in a separate bowl. Add the dry ingredients to the wet mix and combine. Use 24 cupcake liners to line your cupcake baking trays and divide the batter between them. Bake for about 18-20 minutes then remove from the tray and cool on wire racks.

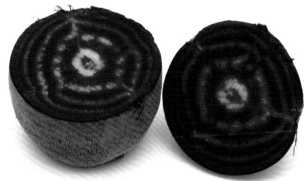

Snacks

Veggie crisps with peanut dip

Ingredients

3 medium beetroots
2 medium potatoes
1 sweet potato
2 tbsp canola oil
For the dip
2 tsp canola oil
1 medium onion
1 clove of garlic, crushed
50g freshly ground peanut butter
1 tsp salt-reduced soy sauce
1 tbsp clear honey
1/2 tsp ground coriander
1/2 tsp ground cumin
Squeeze of lemon juice

Method

For the dip, heat the oil in a pan over medium heat and add the finely diced onion and garlic. Cook for about 4 minutes. Add the coriander and cumin and after about 20 seconds, add the peanut butter, honey, soy sauce and 4 tablespoons of water. Cook over a low heat, stirring regularly, until everything is combined. Put in a small dipping bowl and cover it. For the veggie crisps, pre-heat your oven to 220 degrees Celsius. Slice the vegetables into very thin 2mm slices and put the beetroot in a separate bowl to the potato and sweet potato. Lightly toss the vegetables in the canola oil then spread them on baking sheets lined, with baking paper, in a single layer. Bake for about 35 minutes, turning the veg often, until the potatoes are crisp and golden and the beetroot is moist but firm. Cool on a wire rack.

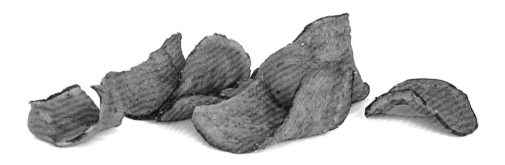

Dippy vegetable crudités

Ingredients

450g of an assortment of firm vegetables, including chopped up celery sticks, baby carrots, capsicum strips, broccoli florets, baby corn (blanched for 1 minute in boiling water), snow peas or green beans (blanched for one minute)

For tomato dip

50g sundried tomatoes (excess oil removed by patting with paper towel)
80g low-fat natural yoghurt
80g low-fat cottage cheese
3/4 cup fresh basil
Freshly-cracked black pepper

For pesto dip

250g low-fat natural yoghurt
1 cup fresh basil
1 tablespoon pine nuts
1 clove of garlic, crushed
Freshly-cracked black pepper

Method

Chop the vegetables that require chopping into sticks and blanch those that need blanching in boiling water for 1 minute. For the tomato dip, cover the sundried tomatoes with boiling water and cover them, then leave them for about 30 minutes to rehydrate. Drain them well and use a paper towel to pat them dry before chopping them finely. In a food processor, puree the yoghurt and cottage cheese, then transfer to a bowl. Stir through the chopped tomatoes then cover and chill until ready to serve. For the pesto dip, puree the basil, pine nuts and garlic in a blender until it has a paste consistency. Add the yoghurt one spoonful at a time until well combined. Season with pepper, cover and then chill in a refrigerator until ready to serve.

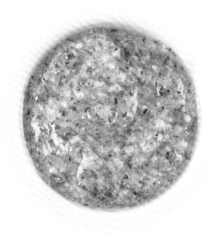

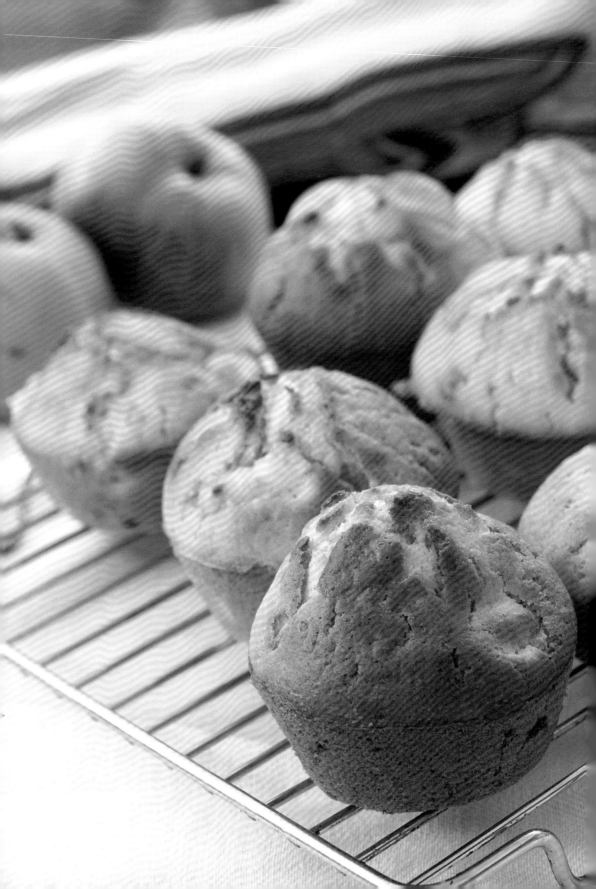

Sweet apple, almond and carrot muffins with bran

Ingredients

3/4 cup chopped apple (Granny Smith, Pink Lady)
3/4 cup grated carrot
1/2 cup slivered almonds
1 cup wholemeal flour
1/4 cup brown sugar
2 cups all-bran cereal
2 tbsp clear honey
2 egg whites
3/4 cup reduced-fat milk
1/2 cup unsweetened apple sauce
1 1/4 tsp baking soda
1 tsp cinnamon
1/4 tsp salt

Method

Pre-heat your oven to 180 degrees Celsius. In a large bowl, mix together the all-bran cereal, flour, brown sugar, almonds, baking soda, cinnamon and salt. In a different bowl, mix together the honey, egg whites, milk and apple sauce, then add the wet mixture into a well at the centre of the bowl of dry ingredients. Mix together well until the mixture is no longer wet. Fold through the chopped apple and grated carrots. Bake for between 20 and 25 minutes. Cool on a wire rack.

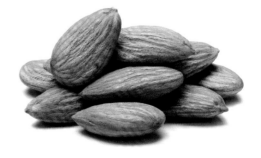

Drinks

Wake-up drink

Ingredients
Boiling water
1/2 lemon and juice

Method
It doesn't get any easier than this. Boil some water, then add to it half a sliced lemon and the juice of the remaining half. Substitute this drink for your morning tea or coffee. It stimulates your metabolism, is a great detoxifier and is great for your skin. Add a little honey if you can't handle the sourness.

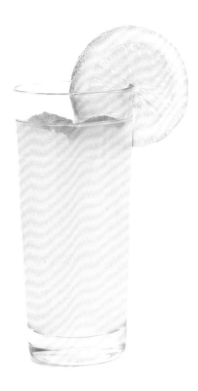

Pomegranate and hibiscus iced tea

Ingredients
1 cup of pomegranate juice
1/4 cup loose hibiscus tea or 12 hibiscus tea herbal bags
4 cups boiling water
4 cups cold water
Juice of 1/2 lemon
Lemon wedges to garnish

Method
Steep the tea or tea bags in boiling water for 3 to 5 minutes, then strain the tea and pour into a large jug. Stir through the pomegranate juice and cold water. Add the lemon juice to help preserve the flavonoids once refrigerated. Refrigerate for at least two hours and serve over ice and the lemon wedges.

Acknowledgements

I am truly grateful to Professor Ian Meredith for the time that he gave me and for the information he generously shared. He has an amazing ability to make the most difficult of concepts easy to understand and his passion to make a difference is inspiring. To Janine Fahri, whose wealth of knowledge was invaluable in the writing of this book, a huge thanks. It's easy to see why you are held in such high esteem within your industry. I am also grateful for the printed and online resources of a number of leading heart organisations from around the world, including The Heart Foundation Australia, The American Heart Association, The British Heart Foundation, the World Health Organisation and The Mayo Clinic. And finally, to my husband Jason and our three little treasures, who fill my heart with love and joy every day.

Professor Ian Meredith AM BSc(Hons), MBBS(Hons), PhD, FRACP, FACC, FCSANZ, FSCAI

Professor Ian Meredith is the Director of MonashHeart, Monash Health and Professor of Cardiology for Monash University in Melbourne, Australia. He is also Executive Director of the Monash Cardiovascular Research Centre, Monash Health, and a member of the board of the National Heart Foundation Victorian branch in Australia. Professor Meredith has more than 20 years experience as a clinical and interventional cardiologist, has performed over 10,000 invasive cardiac and coronary procedures and has been chief investigator or principal investigator for over 30 major international multicentre, randomised trials. In 2012, Professor Meredith was awarded a Member of the Order of Australia for service to medicine in the field of cardiology.

Janine Fahri BSc (Hons) MBANT CNHC

Founder of NutriLife Clinic in Central London, Janine Fahri is a leading nutrition and lifestyle expert with BSc (Hons) degrees in both nutritional therapy and psychology. Adopting a practical and caring approach, Janine devises personal nutrition and lifestyle programmes tailored to suit individual needs. Janine also presents seminars to the general public and corporate sector on a variety of topics including healthy eating, weight loss and stress management. In addition to her private practice, Janine works alongside consultant neurosurgeons and their team in Harley Street and she lectures to the medical profession on specialised subjects including inflammation, digestive dysfunction and drug-nutrient interactions.

Index